GOOD PRACTICES IN ASIA

Effective paradigm shifts towards an improved national response to drugs and HIV/AIDS

SCALE-UP OF HARM REDUCTION IN MALAYSIA

Kuala Lumpur
March 2011

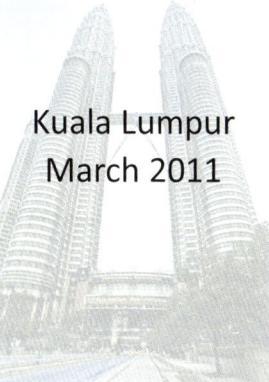

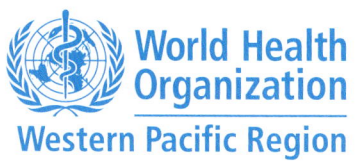

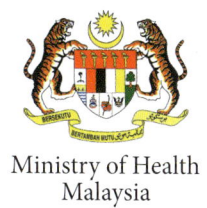

Ministry of Health
Malaysia

WORLD HEALTH ORGANIZATION, WESTERN PACIFIC REGIONAL OFFICE
AND WORLD HEALTH ORGANIZATION OFFICE OF THE REPRESENTATIVE FOR
BRUNEI DARUSSALAM, MALAYSIA AND SINGAPORE

WHO Library Cataloguing in Publication Data

Good practices in Asia : effective paradigm shifts towards an improved national response to drugs and HIV/AIDS : scale-up of harm reduction in Malaysia.

1. HIV infections – prevention and control. 2. Harm reduction. 3. Acquired immunodeficiency syndrome – prevention and control. 4. Drug users. 5. Malaysia

ISBN 978 92 9061 519 4   (NLM Classification: WC 503.6)

© **World Health Organization 2011**

All rights reserved. Publications of the World Health Organization can be obtained from WHO Press, World Health Organization, 20 Avenue Appia, 1211 Geneva 27, Switzerland (tel.: +41 22 791 3264; fax: +41 22 791 4857; e-mail: bookorders@who.int). Requests for permission to reproduce or translate WHO publications – whether for sale or for noncommercial distribution – should be addressed to WHO Press, at the above address (fax: +41 22 791 4806; e-mail: permissions@who.int). For WHO Western Pacific Regional Publications, request for permission to reproduce should be addressed to the Publications Office, World Health Organization, Regional Office for the Western Pacific, P.O. Box 2932, 1000, Manila, Philippines, (fax: +632 521 1036, e-mail: publications@wpro.who.int).

The designations employed and the presentation of the material in this publication do not imply the expression of any opinion whatsoever on the part of the World Health Organization concerning the legal status of any country, territory, city or area or of its authorities, or concerning the delimitation of its frontiers or boundaries. Dotted lines on maps represent approximate border lines for which there may not yet be full agreement.

The mention of specific companies or of certain manufacturers' products does not imply that they are endorsed or recommended by the World Health Organization in preference to others of a similar nature that are not mentioned. Errors and omissions excepted, the names of proprietary products are distinguished by initial capital letters.

All reasonable precautions have been taken by the World Health Organization to verify the information contained in this publication. However, the published material is being distributed without warranty of any kind, either expressed or implied. The responsibility for the interpretation and use of the material lies with the reader. In no event shall the World Health Organization be liable for damages arising from its use.

Printed in Manila

Cover photograph: Shutterstock. *Photographs courtesy*: Communications Team, Malaysian AIDS Council; Dr Norsiah binti Ali and Dr Dharmananda Selvaretnam.

The photographs in this material are used for illustrative purposes only; they do not imply any particular health status, attitudes, behaviours, or actions on the part of any person who appears in the photographs.

TABLE OF CONTENTS

Acronyms	v
Acknowledgements	vii
Foreword	ix
Executive Summary	**11**
1. Introduction	**15**
Malaysia's response to drugs and HIV	17
National drug policy context	20
2. Implementation of harm reduction in Malaysia	**23**
Opioid substitution therapy (OST)	24
Needle and syringe programmes (NSP)	29
Antiretroviral treatment (ART) for people who use drugs (PWUD)	33
Sexual transmission among PWUD	35
Interventions in closed settings	37
3. Analysis of cross-cutting themes	**41**
Communication and advocacy	42
Health systems and human resources	43
Partnerships	44
4. Conclusions and Recommendations	**49**
Conclusions: elements of good practice	50
Recommendations	54

Members of the Technical Working Group

DR SHA'ARI BIN NGADIMAN, Ministry of Health, Malaysia
DR FAZIDAH BINTI YUSWAN, Ministry of Health, Malaysia
DR NORSIAH BINTI ALI, Ministry of Health, Malaysia
DR KHALIJAH BINTI YUSOFF, Ministry of Health, Malaysia
DR FABIO MESQUITA, WHO Western Pacific Regional Office
DR CORINNE CAPUANO, WHO Representative Office for Brunei Darussalam, Malaysia and Singapore
DR HARPAL SINGH, WHO Representative Office for Brunei Darussalam, Malaysia and Singapore
MR PASCAL TANGUAY, Consultant for WHO

Acronyms

AIDS	acquired immune deficiency syndrome
AMAM	Addiction Medicine Association of Malaysia
ANPUD	Asian Network of People who Use Drugs
ASEAN	Association of Southeast Asian Nations
ART	antiretroviral therapy
ATS	amphetamine-type stimulants
BBV	bloodborne virus
DIC	drop-in centre
DOTS	directly observed treatment, short-course
FPMPAM	Federation of Private Medical Practitioners' Association, Malaysia
GP	general practitioner
HBV	hepatitis B virus
HCV	hepatitis C virus
HIV	human immunodeficiency virus
HR3	harm reduction, human rights and human resources (project)
HRWG	Harm Reduction Working Group
M&E	monitoring and evaluation
MAC	Malaysian AIDS Council
MARP	most-at-risk population
MDG	Millennium Development Goal
MMT	methadone maintenance therapy
MOH	Ministry of Health
MOHA	Ministry of Home Affairs
NADA	National Anti-Drugs Agency
NGO	nongovernmental organization
NSP	needle and syringe programme
NTFHR	National Task Force on Harm Reduction
OST	opioid substitution therapy
PLHIV	people living with HIV
PT	PT Foundation (previously known as Pink Triangle)
PWID	people who inject drugs
PWUD	people who use drugs
RM	Malaysian ringgit
SIDA	Swedish International Development Agency
SOP	standard operating procedure

STI	sexually transmitted infection
TB	tuberculosis
UMCAS	University Malaya Centre for Addiction Sciences
UNGASS	United Nations General Assembly Special Session (on HIV/AIDS)
UMMC	University Malaya Medical Centre
UN	United Nations
UNAIDS	Joint United Nations Programme on HIV/AIDS
USD	US dollar
WHO	World Health Organization
WPRO	Regional Office for the Western Pacific

Acknowledgements

This monograph is the result of a series of site visits coupled with key stakeholder interviews. In addition, extensive review was done of the available published literature and documents capturing the experiences of the scale-up of harm reduction in Malaysia. WHO would like to thank all those who shared their opinions, data and materials for the preparation of this report.

Since the integration of harm reduction in the National strategic plan on HIV/AIDS 2006–2010, the Ministry of Health and other national agencies have played a central role in mobilizing local government authorities, local health services, peer outreach workers, other community-based collaborators and relevant sectors including public security to deliver HIV prevention services to people who use drugs, particularly those who inject drugs. Notably, the expansion of needle and syringe programmes and methadone maintenance therapy has been dramatic over the past five years. Preparation of this document would not have been possible without the dedicated work of these institutions and individuals.

This monograph was developed under the leadership of Dr Fabio Mesquita, Technical Officer, Harm Reduction, HIV/AIDS and STI, WHO Regional Office for the Western Pacific (WPRO) and Dr Harpal Singh, Technical Officer, Office of the WHO Representative for Brunei Darussalam, Malaysia and Singapore with the support of Dr Corinne Capuano, WHO Representative for Brunei Darussalam, Malaysia and Singapore. In particular, Dr Mesquita and Dr Singh provided critical conceptual support in the design of the project report while Mr Pascal Tanguay, WHO consultant, provided essential writing and editing inputs.

We express our thanks to peers for their voluntary work. These include Adeeba Kamarulzaman, Center of Excellence for Research in AIDS (CERiA), Malaysia; Alex Wodak, International Harm Reduction Association (IHRA); Anne Bergenstrom, United Nations Regional Task Force (UNRTF); Dean Lewis, Asian Network of People who Use Drugs (ANPUD); Kah Sin Cho, Joint United Nations Programme on HIV/AIDS (UNAIDS); Mahmood Nazar, National Anti-Drug Agency (NADA), Malaysia; Zaman Khan, Malaysian AIDS Council (MAC), Malaysia; and Raymond Tai, Pink Triangle (PT) Foundation, Malaysia; Parimelazhagan Ellan, MAC, Malaysia; Jenithaa S, MAC, Malaysia; and Azahari, MAC, Malaysia.

Sustained, consistent efforts of and support provided by Dato' Dr Hasan bin Abdul Rahman, Director-General of Health; Dr Lokman Hakim bin Suleiman, Director of Disease Control; Dr Sha'ari bin Ngadiman, Head of AIDS/STD Sector, Disease Control

Division, Ministry of Health, Malaysia, to the deployment and implementation of harm reduction services have paved the way for this report.

We also acknowledge the support provided by and efforts of Dato' Dr Zuraidah binti Haji Mohamed, Director-General, National Anti-Drugs Agency, Malaysia towards the timely production of this report.

Special and sincere appreciation goes to the Swedish International Development Agency (SIDA) for their generous financial assistance in publishing this report through the "Harm reduction, human rights, human resources" (HR3) Project.

This document was edited by Bandana Malhotra, and designed and typeset by Netra Shyam.

Foreword

Injecting drug use and sex work have largely driven HIV epidemics in many Asian countries, though transmission has followed different patterns according to the local context. The development of the Malaysian response to HIV and drugs has been timely and coordinated, and its overall implementation has been grounded in scientific evidence, and recognition of the value of multisectoral partnerships and political leadership.

In 2005, the Minister of Health's public announcement outlining the national commitment to rapidly address HIV transmission led to the launch of the first pilot methadone maintenance therapy (MMT) project in October and, shortly thereafter, the implementation of its first needle and syringe programme (NSP) in early 2006. The experience acquired since then and lessons learned through this critical process have been commendable. The endorsement of harm reduction by supportive and committed leadership has been remarkable, in that effective harm reduction interventions have been systematically expanded and integrated into public health services. Government leadership and sustained partnerships with other government and nongovernment agencies have indeed proven to be a key element of Malaysia's success. While challenges remain, the consistent evolution of and progress in the national response to HIV and drugs have been encouraging, and successfully mobilized large numbers of dedicated and committed individuals and groups.

The World Health Organization (WHO) and Ministry of Health (MOH) in Malaysia are therefore committed to sustaining such efforts, which have also been articulated in WHO's *Malaysia Country Cooperation Strategy 2009–2013*. The third Country Cooperation Strategy for Malaysia covers two strategic approaches or "arms". The first arm encompasses WHO's support to Malaysia in selected national health priorities, in tandem with WHO's support to Malaysia's contributions to regional and international health collaboration as part of the second arm. The second arm includes Malaysia's rich experience in harm reduction.

The present document is aligned with the *Strategy to halt and reverse the HIV epidemic among people who inject drugs in Asia and the Pacific 2010–2015* proposed by WHO and recently developed jointly by the UN Regional Task Force on Injecting Drug Use, WHO and other UN agencies and partners. The strategy represents a "call for action" designed to provide practical tools – such as this document – for use by national governments and other agencies to guide the strategic planning process and service delivery. In this respect, Malaysia's efforts to scale down compulsory drug treatment and develop comprehensive harm reduction services are elements of good practice that deserve to be highlighted.

The fascinating examples described in this monograph remind us of the leadership principles, the value of community participation and the need for multisectoral collaboration and coordination, as outlined in the Regional strategy.

Dato' Dr Hasan bin Abdul Rahman
Director-General of Health,
Ministry of Health, Malaysia.

Dr Corinne Capuano
WHO Representative for Brunei Darussalam,
Malaysia and Singapore

EXECUTIVE SUMMARY

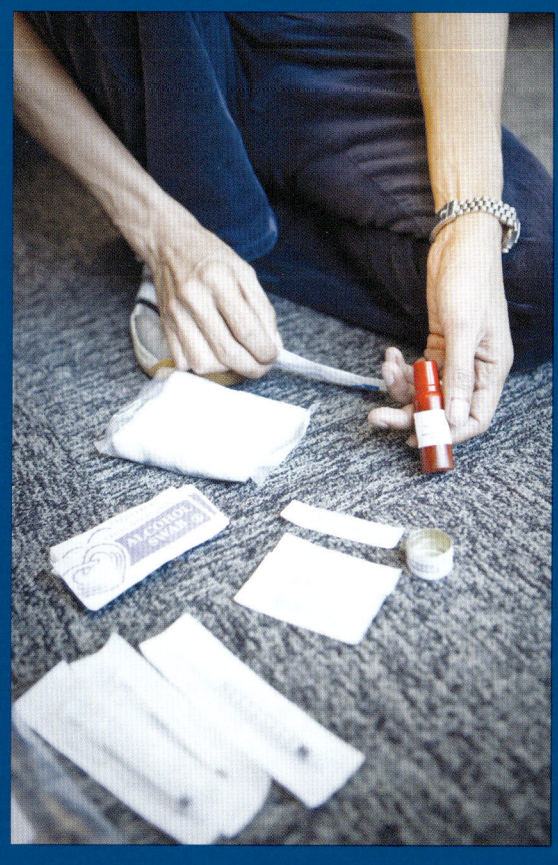

Executive summary

The spread of HIV in Malaysia, though not fully contained, has been on the decline over the past decade, from 7000 new cases recorded in 2002 to just over 3000 cases in 2009. Despite considerable efforts to curb HIV/AIDS transmission in Malaysia, HIV remains a national priority. The World Health Organization (WHO) qualifies Malaysia's epidemic as "concentrated": low rates of infection in the general population, as evidenced by an estimated adult HIV prevalence of 0.4%, and seemingly isolated high prevalence rates among high-risk groups such as people who inject drugs (PWID), prison inmates and female sex workers.

Since the inception of pilot harm reduction projects around 2005, needle and syringe programmes (NSPs) and particularly methadone maintenance therapy (MMT) have remained at the heart of the national response to drugs and HIV/AIDS. In addition, the Malaysian harm reduction programme remains the cornerstone of the national HIV prevention strategy, which is almost entirely funded by the Malaysian government, though some technical assistance has been systematically provided by WHO. Implemented in partnership with nongovernmental organizations (NGOs) and private health practitioners, it is a better-funded programme among all the national HIV prevention activities.

The integration of harm reduction has been widely accepted as an important landmark in the government's change of attitude towards drug use in Malaysia. Indeed, the paradigm shift from a repressive approach to drugs relying on punishment and law enforcement action, to an approach that now fully integrates and accepts public health imperatives implemented in collaboration with health professionals and law enforcement officers has been documented and recognized as an important success for the country and the Region as a whole.

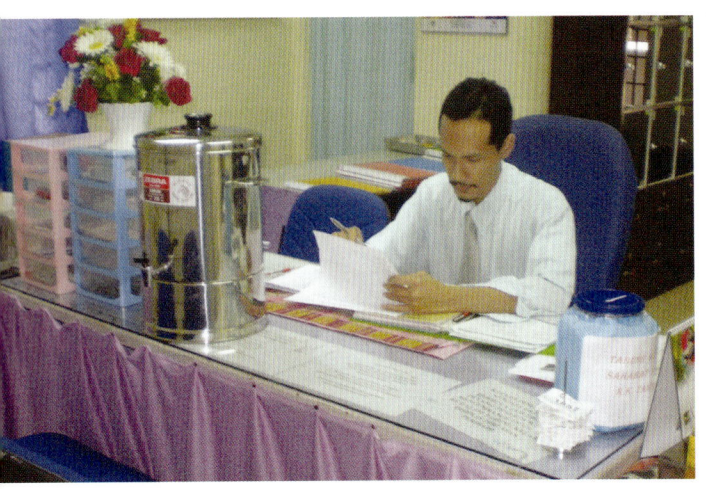

Another paradigm shift is currently taking place under the extraordinary leadership of key individuals and agencies. Where the Malaysian government has moved from a repressive approach to an approach integrating health imperatives a few years ago, key agencies are again shifting programmatic objectives from compulsory abstinence to voluntary treatment options.

At this point in time, it is particularly relevant to review the successes achieved in Malaysia with regard to the implementation of harm reduction services. Given the assertion above of a double paradigm shift in a short span of time, this report verifies and documents the process through which these shifts have occurred. By doing so, it will become possible to identify the key elements contributing to the success of the national harm reduction programme in Malaysia and also identify the gaps and challenges for the future of the response.

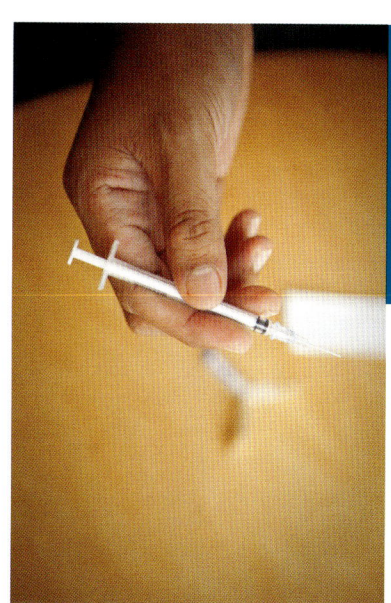

The shift is also being reflected in an increasing range of available health and social care services, as well as their integration with other health systems already in place in Malaysia. The provision of MMT and antiretroviral therapy (ART) in one location, particularly in closed institutions, also lends weight to the proposition of an emerging paradigm. With an expanded range of such institutions providing health and social care services for people who use drugs (PWUD) – whether they be delivered through hospitals, district health clinics, NGO-operated drop-in centres (DICs), prisons and other closed institutions, and mosques – access to health-care service options in Malaysia has been systematically increasing. Indeed, the range of services offered at each site is also increasing rapidly, from virtually no harm reduction services in 2005 to a full-fledged national programme within five years. This emerging paradigm is an important element of good practice, given a decreased reliance on compulsory treatment centres as well as a more sensitized and evidence-based response to the needs of PWUD.

Other elements of good practice include the rapid scale-up of a comprehensive range of harm reduction services made available through a variety of outlets and settings; deployment of effective policies and procedures to guide implementation and monitoring and evaluation (M&E) of programmes; accreditation and registration of service providers as well as parallel training and capacity building; allocation of significant proportions of the national budget to support implementation; excellent collaboration, communication and partnerships between the stakeholders involved in the national response to drugs and HIV/AIDS; high-level commitment and support from key agencies from various sectors; and integration of harm reduction services into existing health systems.

In contrast, certain components of the national response need to be addressed. These include human resource capacity across all interventions, revision and development of standard operating procedures (SOPs) for each intervention in the comprehensive harm reduction package, the need for rapid scale-up of coverage of

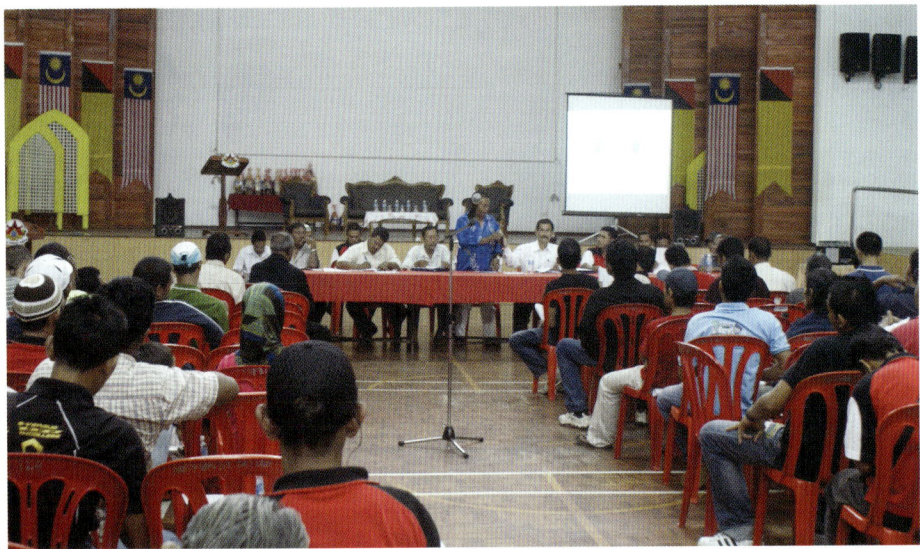

key interventions, especially counselling and condom distribution, harmonization of laws with existing practices and decisions in the country, as well as the development of a national communication strategy to accompany the next national strategic plan on HIV/AIDS.

Overall, it is clear that though Malaysia's response does need some further investments, it already incorporates several elements of good practice that support effective harm reduction among PWUD. The preponderance of these elements of good practice distinguishes Malaysia's response to drugs and HIV/AIDS from that of its neighbours, and can be presented as an important Asian model for further advocacy and scale-up of harm reduction services.

1 Introduction

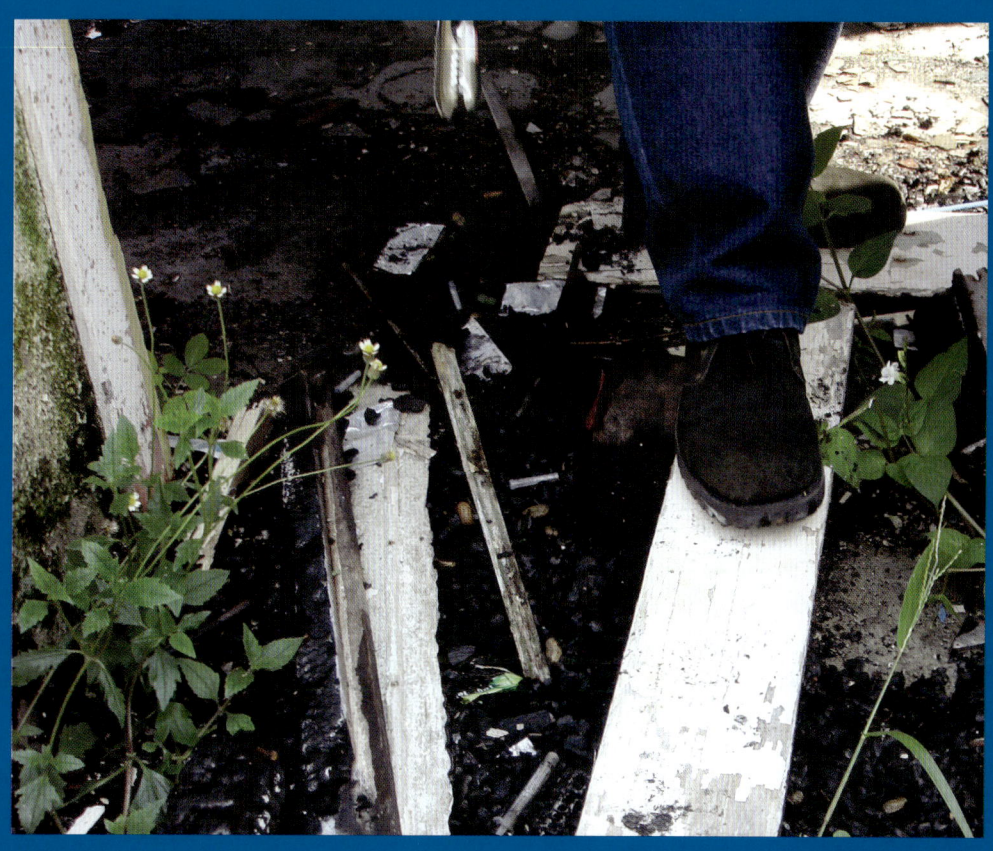

Introduction

A considerable number of people inject drugs in Asia, representing approximately 25% of all people who inject drugs (PWID) worldwide.[1] Though the average Regional HIV prevalence among PWID is 16%, countries such as Malaysia have recorded over half of all PWID to be living with HIV.[1] In Malaysia, the first case of HIV was officially detected in 1986. From then till 2009, a total of 87 710 cases were officially detected, of which 15 317 had AIDS. A total of 13 394 AIDS-related deaths have since been recorded, leaving 74 316 people living with HIV (PLHIV).

Injecting drug use has been reported in 24 countries in Asia. Among these countries, only 15 have implemented needle and syringe programmes (NSPs) to some extent or the other, and only 12 provide opioid substitution therapy (OST). Up to 65% of the countries in Asia recently reported targeted antiretroviral treatment (ART) for PWID.[2] Civil society groups operate many of these services with little training or capacity, and raids by law enforcement agencies at delivery sites continue to hamper effective interventions. Despite the best efforts and investments in the Region, coverage of harm reduction services among most-at-risk PWID remains largely insufficient to impact national prevalence rates.[1]

The World Health Organization Regional Office for the Western Pacific (WHO WPRO) comprises 37 countries from the Mekong River Valley in Asia to countries in the Pacific. Many of the epidemics in the Region are currently driven by needle-sharing and drug use. The HIV epidemic in countries such as China, Malaysia and Viet Nam is largely driven by injecting drug use. Comprehensive responses to HIV and drug use in the Region are being defined and implemented in Cambodia, Lao People's Democratic Republic, Malaysia and the Philippines. The other 31 countries are considered to have a very low prevalence (except Papua New Guinea, which has a generalized epidemic, though transmission vectors are almost exclusively related to sex).[3]

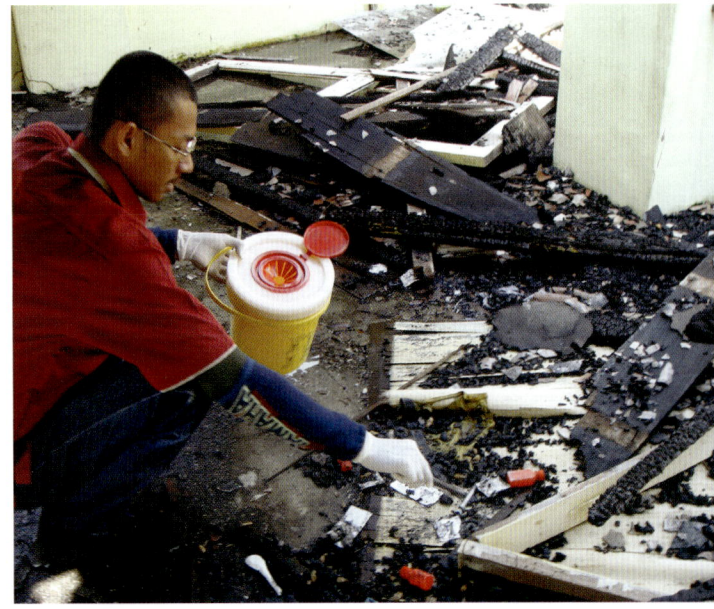

....

1 International Harm Reduction Association (IHRA). *Global state of harm reduction*. London, IHRA, 2010.
2 Burnet Institute. *Harm reduction in Asia: progress towards universal access to harm reduction services among people who inject drugs*. Melbourne, Burnet Institute, 2010.
3 Mesquita F et al. Accelerating harm reduction interventions to confront the HIV epidemic in the Western Pacific and Asia: the role of WHO (WPRO). *Harm Reduction Journal*, 2008, 5:26.

Figure 1. HIV, AIDS and deaths related to HIV/AIDS, Malaysia 1986–2010

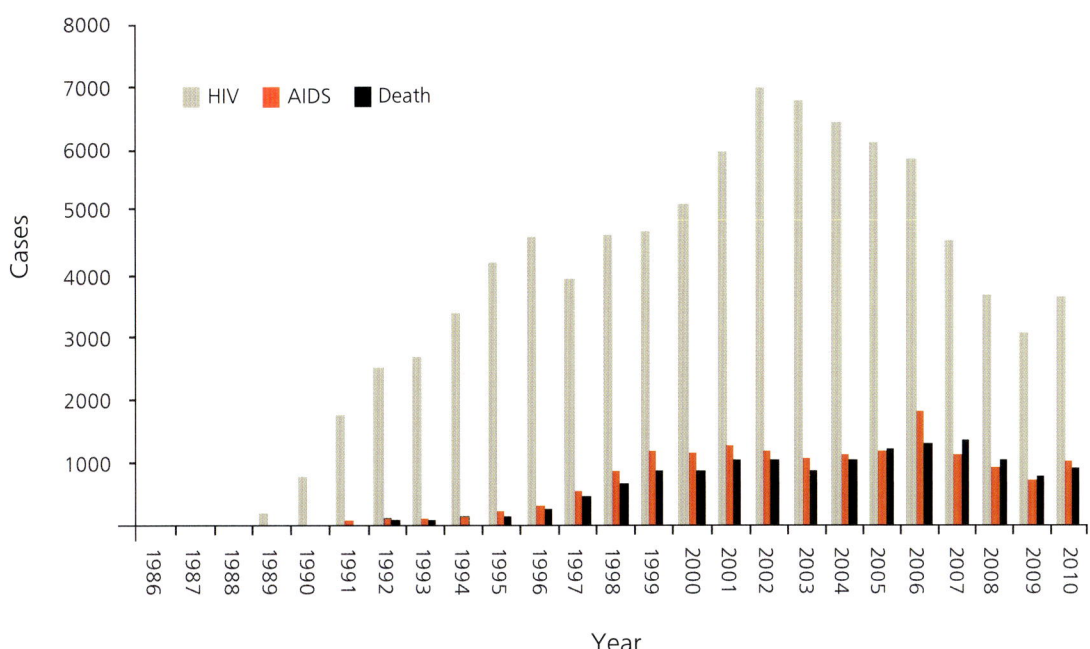

Malaysia's response to drugs and HIV

Nearly 80 000 people are currently living with HIV/AIDS in Malaysia.[4] After the first case of HIV was detected in 1986, a general consensus has since been arrived at, which acknowledges injecting drug use as one of the key drivers of the HIV epidemic in Malaysia. In 2009, out of the average nine new HIV cases recorded every day, six would have contracted HIV through injecting drug use, and three via sexual transmission.[5]

In contrast, the total number of PWID in Malaysia is estimated at around 170 000 with an HIV prevalence of 22.1%.[4] However, this number is likely to be a conservative estimate and additional persons using, but not necessarily injecting, drugs are at increased risk for HIV transmission. To make matters more difficult, among PWID, existing data point to a prevalence of hepatitis C virus (HCV) of nearly 90%.[6]

The Declaration of Commitment on HIV/AIDS adopted by the United Nations General Assembly Special Session on HIV/AIDS (UNGASS) in 2001, to which Malaysia was a signatory, called on all Member States to make available a wide range of prevention

---

4 Ministry of Health. *Malaysia UNGASS country progress report*. Kuala Lumpur, MOH, 2010.
5 MoH. *National strategic plan on HIV/AIDS 2006–2010*. Kuala Lumpur, MOH, 2005.
6 Vicknasingham B et al. 2009. Prevalence rates and risk factors for hepatitis C among drug users not in treatment in Malaysia. *Drug and Alcohol Review*, 2009, 28:447–454.

Figure 2. Reported HIV infections by major risk categories, 1986–2010

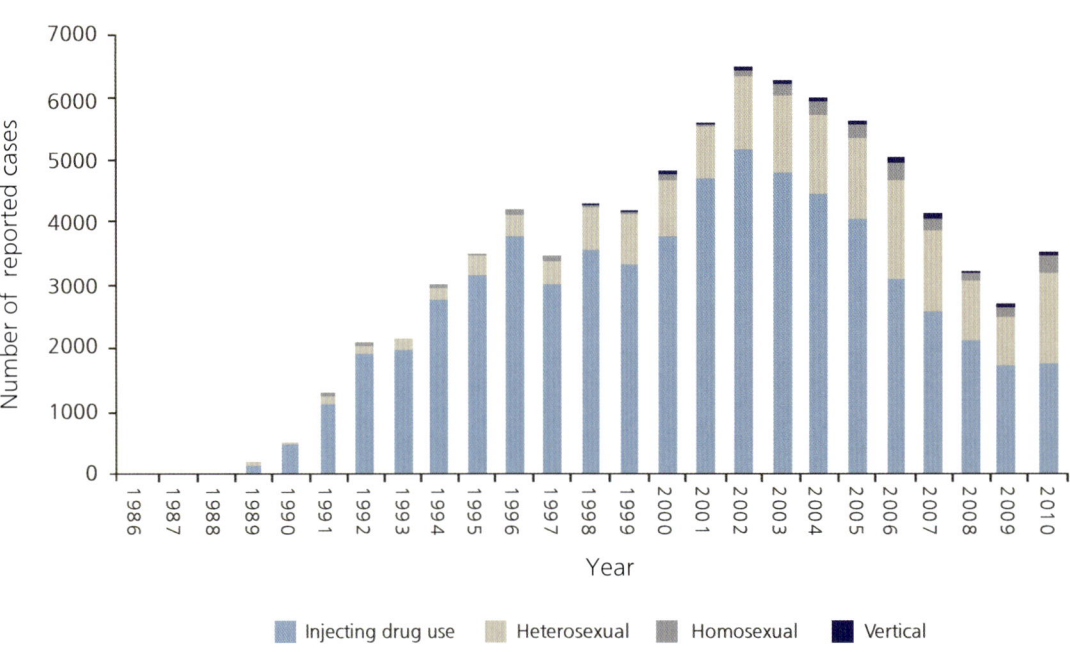

programmes including harm reduction efforts related to drug use. The fact that Malaysia has been able to achieve all but one of the eight mid-term Millennium Development Goals (MDGs) – the one related to reversal of the HIV epidemic – spurred the government into accepting the need for a different approach in 2005: the Malaysian government incorporated the following in its National strategic plan on HIV/AIDS 2006–2010:

As a key intervention for slowing the growth of the epidemic and preventing transition to a generalized epidemic, the National Strategic Plan promotes a harm reduction approach to reducing HIV vulnerability among injecting drug users. Harm reduction programmes recognize that for many drug users, total abstinence from psychoactive substances is not a practical option. It aims to help drug users reduce their injection frequency in a safe environment.[5]

In the same year, the government launched its harm reduction programme. The first pilot methadone maintenance therapy (MMT) project commenced in 17 centres in nine states, with support from the newly convened National Task Force on Harm Reduction (NTFHR). Four months later, in 2006, the national government implemented three pilot NSPs in Penang, Johor and Kuala Lumpur through local NGOs and subsequently in government health clinics. In 2008, MMT

INTRODUCTION

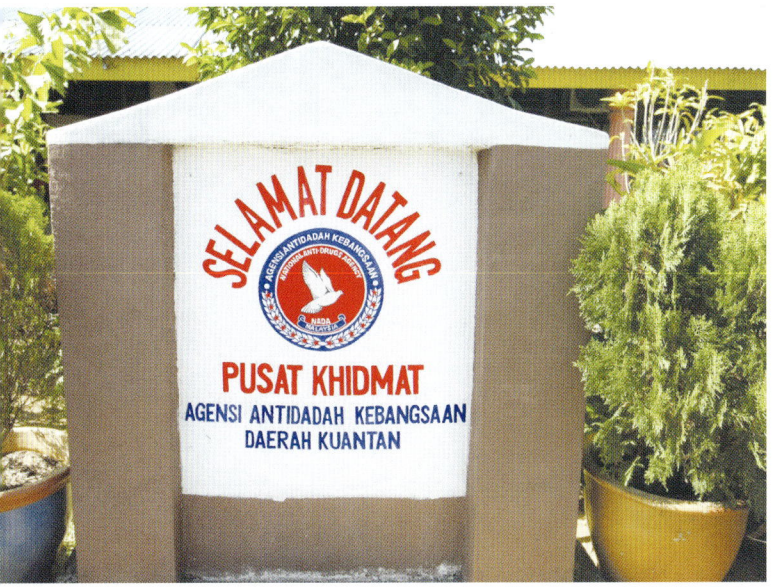

was piloted in closed settings, both in Pengkalan Chepa prison and in three National Anti-Drugs Agency (NADA)-operated aftercare centres as well as in community settings.

All three pilots have been extremely successful, despite the incredible hurdles the national programme has had to overcome to reach current outcomes. Indeed, a mid-term evaluation of the national harm reduction programme conducted by WHO concluded that "Malaysia has moved swiftly from pilot harm reduction projects to a scaled-up response to HIV [among] injecting drug users, a strategy that ties in with the National Strategic Plan on HIV/AIDS for 2006 to 2010 [while recognizing that] the evolution from pilots to institutionalized programmes is not an easy process."[7]

Since the inception of these pilot projects, NSPs and particularly MMT remain at the heart of the national response to drugs and HIV. In addition, the Malaysian harm reduction programme remains the cornerstone of the national HIV prevention strategy. Implemented in partnership with nongovernmental organizations (NGOs) and private health practitioners, it remains the best-funded programme among all the national HIV prevention activities.

With the success of the pilot projects, it was not long before rapid scale-up proceeded across Malaysia. As of June 2010, 211 MMT access points are operational across the country – 37 in government hospitals, 112 in health clinics, 21 in registered private clinics, 24 through NADA-operated community-based aftercare centres, 15 in prison settings as well as in the University Malaya Centre for Addiction Sciences (UMCAS) and Ar-Rahman Mosque. In addition, over 200 general practitioners (GPs) are dispensing methadone and other substitution drugs, covering more than 20 000 patients. Approximately 352 sites are distributing sterile needles and injecting equipment through 267 outreach contact points, 73 government clinics and 12 centres (including three DICs).

The spread of HIV in Malaysia, though not fully contained, has been on the decline over the past decade. From 6978 new cases (28.5 per 100 000 population) recorded

---

7 Lee SS. *Report on an interim review and a gap analysis of the harm reduction programme in Malaysia*. 2007.

in 2002, there were about 3080 cases (10.8 per 100 000 population) in 2009.[4] Despite efforts to curb HIV/AIDS transmission in Malaysia, HIV remains a national priority. WHO qualifies Malaysia's epidemic as "concentrated": low rates of infection in the general population, as evidenced by an estimated adult HIV prevalence of 0.4%, and seemingly isolated high prevalence rates among high-risk groups such as PWID, prison inmates and female sex workers.[8]

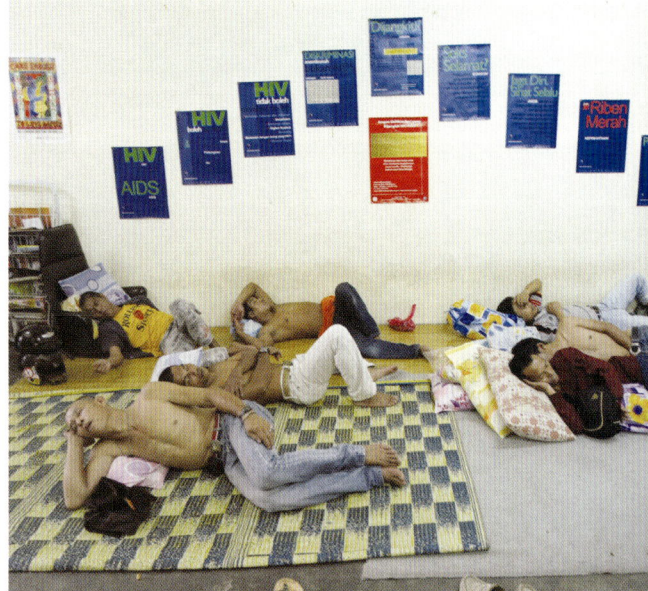

National drug policy context

National commitments to achieving a drug-free Malaysia by 2015 have been signed by the government in the context of the Association of Southeast Asian Nations (ASEAN), which has called for a reinforcement of public security- and law enforcement-driven efforts to reduce drug use and trafficking in the Region. In fact, the Malaysian government's approach to addressing drug use and trafficking, enshrined in the Dangerous Drugs Act, 1952 has revolved around a repressive strategy linked with severe punishment, including corporal punishment.[9,10,11]

In contrast, the Drug Dependants (Treatment and Rehabilitation) Act, 1983 has provided the opportunity to divert those arrested for drug-related crimes to compulsory drug treatment centres.[12] The centres are managed by NADA, under the supervision of the Ministry of Home Affairs (MOHA), in collaboration with the MOH. However, drug-related recidivism inevitably leads to a prison sentence.

Malaysian prisons currently hold 36 040 persons incarcerated in its 31 prisons; the country has a total capacity of 32 000 across 30 prisons. At least 16 other detention centres are in place, including drug treatment centres, illegal immigrants' depots and juvenile institutions.[13] In 2007, 16 237 drug users (or 38% of the prison population)

---

8   Kamarulzaman A. Antiretroviral therapy in Malaysia: identifying barriers to universal access. *Journal of HIV Therapy*, 2009, 3:573–582.
9   Government of Malaysia. *Dangerous Drugs Act, 1952*. Kuala Lumpur, 2006.
10 Lawyers Collective HIV/AIDS Unit. *A preview of law and policy in South and South East Asia – drugs, treatment and harm reduction*. 2010. Available from: http://aidsdatahub.org/en/reference-materials/aids-policies-and-briefs.
11 WHO. *Assessment of compulsory treatment of people who use drugs in Cambodia, China, Malaysia and Viet Nam: an application of selected human rights principles*. Manila, WHO WPRO, 2009. Available at: http://www.who.int/hiv/topics/idu/drug_dependence/compulsory_treatment_wpro.pdf (accessed on 01 March 2011).
12 Laws of Malaysia. *Drug Dependants Treatment and Rehabilitation Act, 1983*. Commissioner of Law Revision, 2006. Available at: http://www.agc.gov.my/Akta/Vol.%206/Act%20283.pdf (accessed on 02 March 2011).
13 International Centre for Prison Studies (ICPS). *Prison brief for Malaysia*. 2010. Available at: http://www.kcl.ac.uk/depsta/law/research/icps/worldbrief/wpb_country.php?country=102 (accessed on 02 March 2011).

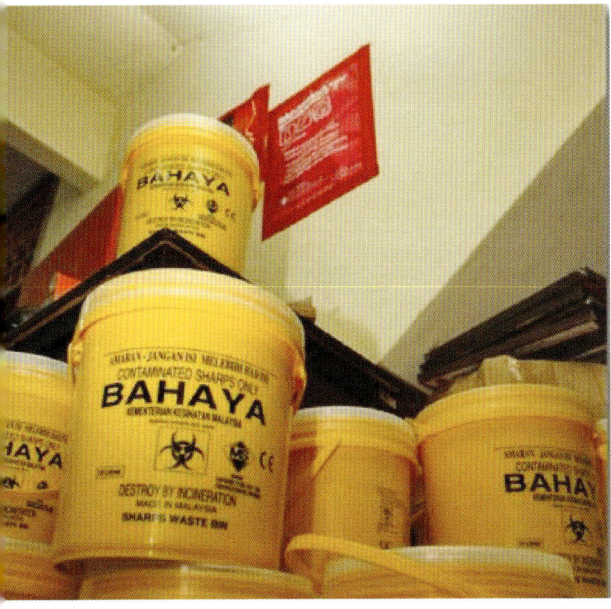

were imprisoned for drug-related offences.[14] Juveniles account for 16.6% of those falling under the jurisdiction of the Dangerous Drugs Act, 1952, particularly for possession and use of drugs.[15] (According to the Prison Act, 1995, a juvenile or a young offender is defined as "a prisoner who is under the age of 21 years".) Though the prison system is still overcrowded, there has been a marked decrease in the population in drug rehabilitation centres across Malaysia. PWUD are increasingly being placed in community-based rehabilitation centres in 93 districts across the country.

The Drug Dependants (Treatment and Rehabilitation) Act, 1983[12] and the integration of harm reduction have been widely accepted as important landmarks in the government's change of attitude towards drug use in Malaysia. Indeed, the paradigm shift from a repressive approach to drugs relying on punishment and law enforcement action to an approach that now fully integrates and accepts public health imperatives implemented collaboratively by health professionals and law enforcement officers has been documented and recognized as an important success for the country and the Region as a whole.

---

14 HIV and AIDS Data Hub for Asia–Pacific. *Law, policy and HIV in Asia and the Pacific: implications on the vulnerability of men who have sex with men, female sex workers and injecting drug users*. 2010. Available at: http://www.aidsdatahub.org/en/regional-profile/law-and-policy (accessed on 02 March 2011).

15 Kassim Abd Wahab Bin. *Juveniles on remand: trends and practices in Malaysia*. Undated. Available at: http://www.unafei.or.jp/english/pdf/RS_No68/No68_17PA_Kassim.pdf (accessed on 02 March 2011).

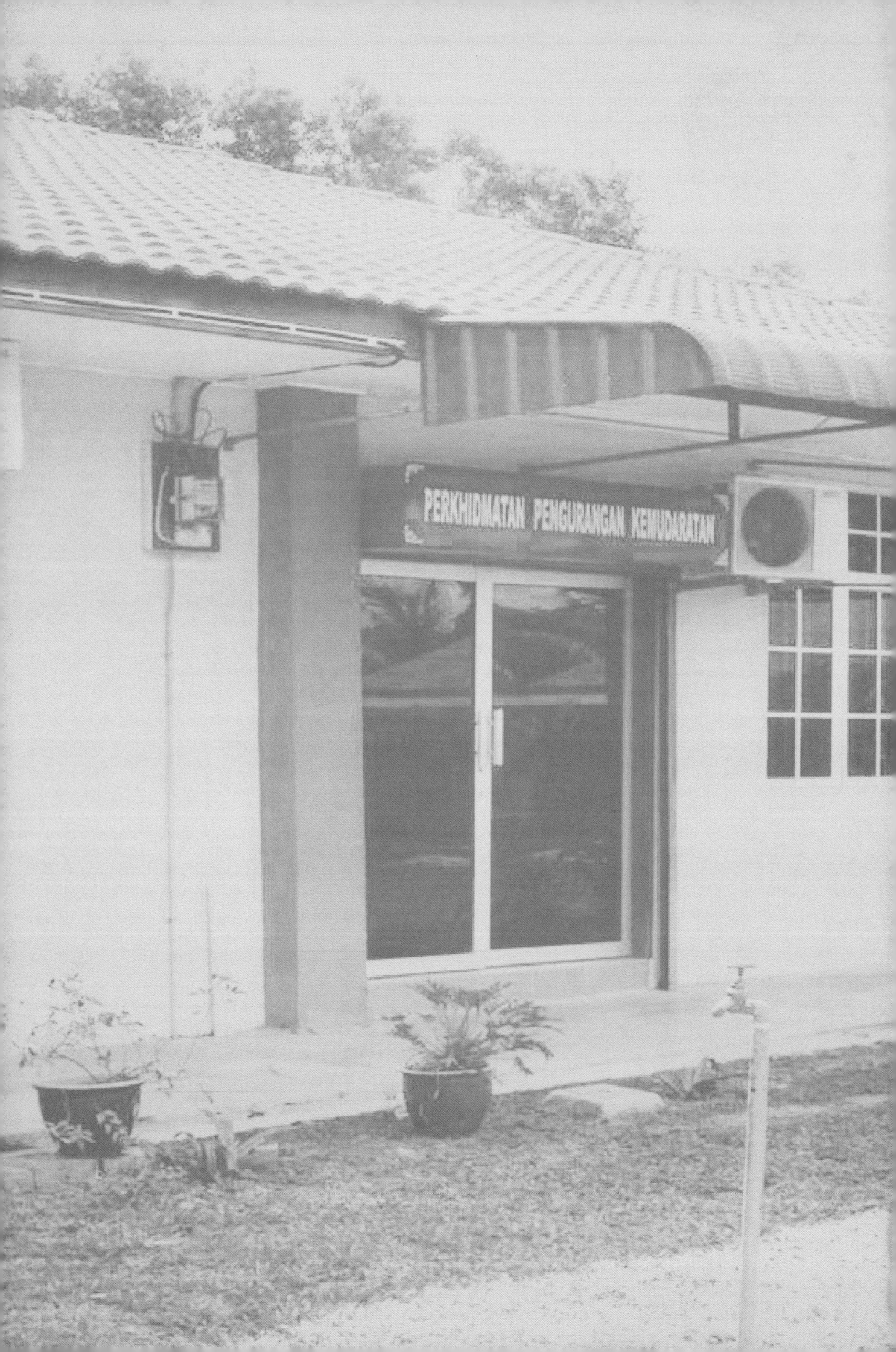

2 Implementation of harm reduction in Malaysia

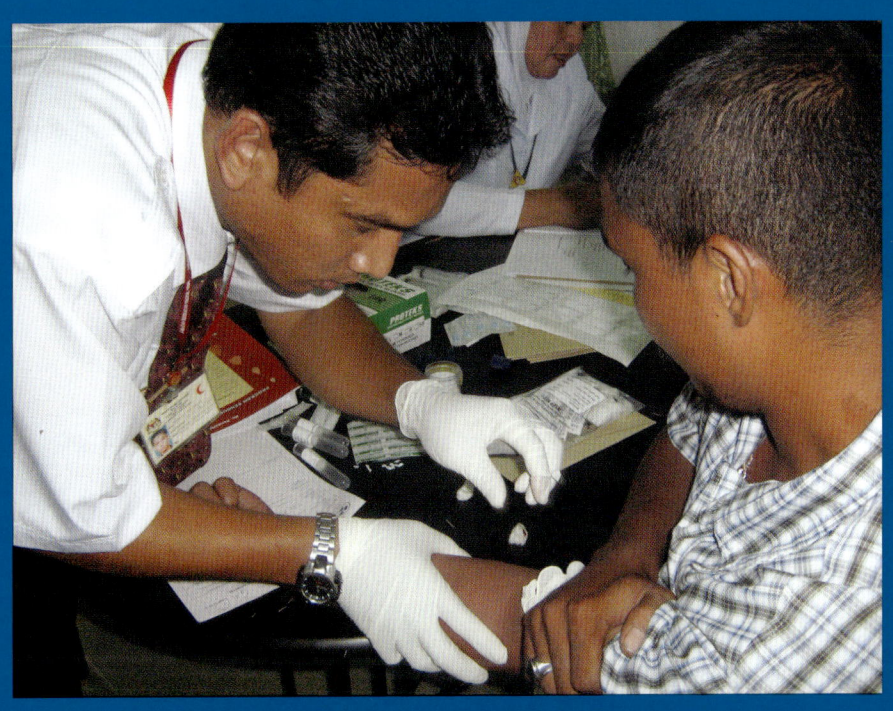

Implementation of harm reduction in Malaysia

The implementation of harm reduction in Malaysia has focused on OST to a large extent and on NSPs as well. However, WHO acknowledges and promotes a comprehensive package of interventions to address HIV prevention, treatment, care and support among PWUD. The comprehensive package includes nine interventions:[16]

Standard operating procedures in Malaysia

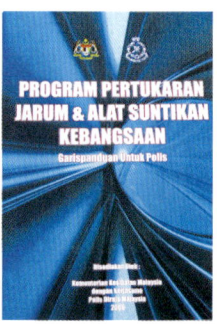 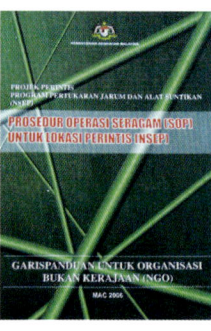 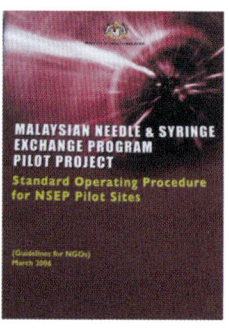 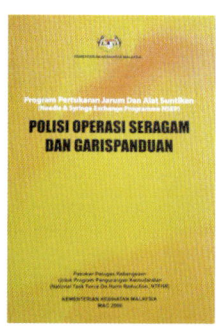

1. Needle and syringe programmes (NSPs)
2. Opioid substitution therapy (OST) and other drug dependence treatment
3. HIV testing and counselling
4. Antiretroviral therapy (ART)
5. Prevention and treatment of sexually transmitted infections (STIs)
6. Condom programmes for PWID and their sexual partners
7. Targeted information, education and communication for PWID and their sexual partners
8. Vaccination for, and diagnosis and treatment of, viral hepatitis
9. Prevention, diagnosis and treatment of tuberculosis (TB).

Although this report focuses on NSP, OST, ART, condom distribution and closed settings, it is important to keep the comprehensive package in mind to confirm the overall good practice elements present in the national response in Malaysia.

Opioid substitution therapy (OST)

As of June 2010, over 13 471 individuals were registered across the country's 211 free MMT service outlets and an additional estimated 20 000 individuals were accessing fee-based OST through private practitioners. Table 1 provides an overview of the growth of MMT access points in Malaysia since the inception of the national harm reduction programme.

---

[16] UNAIDS, UNODC, WHO. *Technical guide for countries to set targets for universal access to HIV prevention, treatment and care for injecting drug users.* Geneva, UNAIDS, 2009.

Table 1: Distribution of MMT access points in Malaysia, 2006–2010 (June)

MMT	2006	2007	2008	2009	2010 (June)
Hospitals	8	25	27	35	40
Government clinics	2	32	32	77	134
Private clinics	7	9	9	14	21
Anti-Drugs Agency	0	0	3	24	25
Prisons	0	0	4	12	18
Others	0	0	0	0	2
Total	17	66	75	162	240

The rapid scale-up of MMT since 2006 has been recognized as a landmark achievement, in large part due to high-level commitment generated through coordinated advocacy efforts. The commitment to scaling-up MMT, based on UN recommendations to achieve 60% coverage of an estimated 170 000 PWID in Malaysia, have led to a rapid increase in coverage and a parallel strengthening, expansion and integration of relevant health systems. Despite falling short of the established targets, as outlined in Table 2, the momentum of MMT service delivery created in Malaysia is impressive when considered with the behind-the-scenes preparation, alignment and systems strengthening that has taken place.

It should be noted that among more than 20 000 registered MMT clients, 66% are actively working in a salaried job. This indicates that MMT services can significantly stabilize an individual's lifestyle, helping the person to maintain social commitments and become a contributing member of society.[17,18]

Table 2: Targets for the number of PWID on MMT treatment, 2006–2010

Year	2006	2007	2008	2009	2010
Targets (number)	1 200	5 000	10 000	15 000	25 000
Expected coverage (%)	1.0	4.2	8.3	12.5	20.8
Actual coverage (%)	0.9	2.9	5.0	6.6	7.9

In the background, diverse modalities of access and key support mechanisms have been deployed and implemented to ensure the success of Malaysia's MMT services. For example, MMT services have been made available in Malaysia through a wide range of service providers, including government-accredited health facilities (hospitals, health clinics, drug treatment centres), private GPs, civil society-operated projects, in closed settings and, more recently, through mosques. *The Review and evaluation on harm reduction programme in Malaysia*[18,19] recognizes that the

---

17 MoH. *Expansion of the harm reduction programme – a report on the national harm reduction up-scaling workshop.* Kuala Lumpur, Ministry of Health, 2009.
18 Wodak A. 2009. *Review of opioid substitution treatment in Malaysia for the World Health Organization.*
19 WHO. *Review and evaluation on harm reduction programme in Malaysia.* Kuala Lumpur, WHO, 2008.

diversity of service outlet options is a strength to be maintained and cultivated in Malaysia's MMT roll-out.

In all cases, and whoever the prescriber of MMT may be, the medical officer in charge of the service outlet must comply with the *National policy on drug substitution therapy*[20] and conform to MOH's *National MMT guidelines.*[21] These documents stipulate the conditions under which methadone can be dispensed to ensure the safety of clients and oversight of the process by outside agencies. For example, the national policy promotes directly observed treatment, short-course

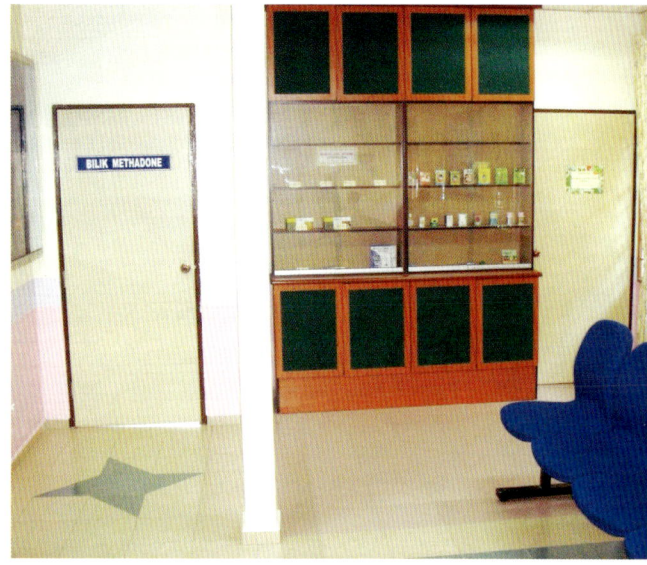

(DOTS) and allows take-away doses only after four to six weeks of compliance with programme guidelines. The policy further compels medical officers to register with national authorities and obtain accreditation through a government-approved workshop based on an academic training module. At the end of 2009, the Addiction Medicine Association of Malaysia (AMAM) and the Federation of Private Medical Practitioners' Association, Malaysia (FPMPAM) reported 631 registered and accredited medical officers in the country.[22]

The policy urges medical officers to collect documentation in order to establish and verify client baseline, treatment and outcomes, including testing for drugs, HIV, HCV and hepatitis B virus (HBV). The national guidelines indicate that provision of pre- and post-test counselling should accompany testing. They also recommend a gradual increase in the daily dose of methadone until optimal levels are reached, generally ending at between 60 and 100 mg, representing an important increase compared to dosage levels in 2006.[18]

Since its inception, the Malaysian MMT programme has documented client satisfaction through application of the WHO Quality of Life tool and other data collection techniques.[18] Results indicate that the MMT services are attractive to clients, which is further confirmed by the high volume of demand for such services.

Access to MMT through government-run programmes has significantly improved and is being provided in diverse locations, from health centres to closed settings (*see* later subsection for details of MMT in closed settings). MMT delivery remains squarely the province and responsibility of medical officers and health officials.

---

20 MOH. *National policy on drug substitution therapy.* Kuala Lumpur, MOH, 2007.
21 MOH. *National methadone maintenance therapy guidelines.* Kuala Lumpur, MOH, 2006.
22 AMAM, FPMPAM. *National drugs substitution treatment report.* Kuala Lumpur, Academy of Medicine Malaysia, 2009.

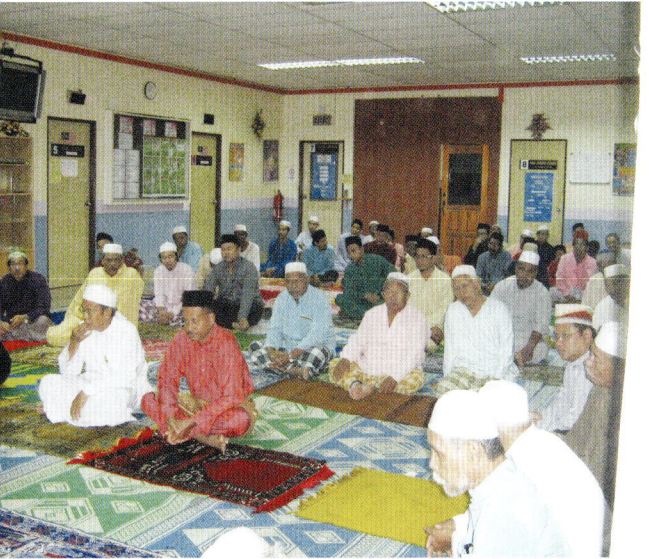

However, the high demand for MMT services has imposed a need to rely heavily on GPs for front-line service provision, an apparent prerequisite to achieving high coverage as demonstrated in other countries.[22]

In private practice, GPs provide suboxone more often than methadone, even though the former is more expensive than the latter and the costs usually increase for the client.[17] GPs have expressed concerns over time management, given that PWUD require close follow up and extensive counselling, as well as financial constraints, should reimbursement from the government be too low to cover their operational costs. Also, accreditation is a common concern across the spectrum of involved stakeholders, although the government, the University Malaya and AMAM have developed accreditation and training modules to scale-up capacity.

In responding to harm reduction, the UMCAS has recently initiated the world's first MMT service operating out of a mosque in Kuala Lumpur. With support from the Federal Territory State Religious Department, the project has been operating since April 2010 out of the Ar-Rahman mosque, reaching out to approximately 50 clients living near a "port" (a shared spaced among PWUD where consumption occurs).

As part of the government strategy, expansion of MMT in closed settings – prisons and drug treatment centres – has been consistent. MMT services in closed settings are detailed in a later section of this report.

In order to put in place the necessary health systems to deliver effective MMT in Malaysia, the MOH had to invest significant resources from its national budget as well as establish strong and value-enhancing partnerships. From the start, Malaysia's national harm reduction programme, including the MMT component, is almost entirely funded by the national government. In 2009, out of the RM 21 million earmarked for the national harm reduction programme, RM 15 million was invested in MMT.

As provided in the *National policy on drug substitution therapy*,[20] elements of the MMT programme operated by the national government as well as private medical officers must be monitored and evaluated in a transparent manner, so that service providers remain accountable for their actions. This is confirmed by the *National drug substitution treatment report*, which clearly states that, "All forms of drug substitution therapy can and must be monitored closely to prevent system failure".[22]

To that effect, MOH has set up its own surveillance information system for monitoring MMT patients. In parallel, AMAM and FPMPAM have set up another national registry for MMT providers as well as GPs operating privately.

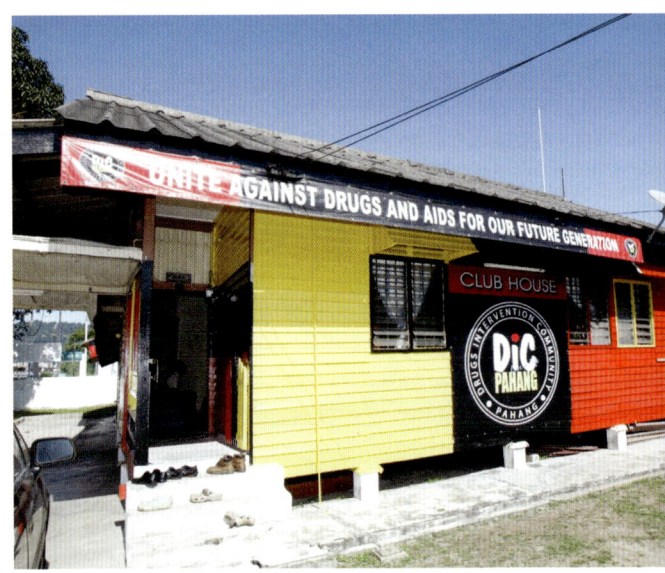

In conclusion, the delivery of MMT in Malaysia can be considered good practice. The several key elements include timely implementation and expansion of services, a service deployment strategy grounded on a health systems approach, multiplication of innovative service access options along with some of the elements of the comprehensive package recommended by UN agencies, effective and transparent partnerships involving all sectors, and a mechanism to track client satisfaction throughout the process. All these are backed by clear and unwavering commitment from high-level individuals and key agencies to the development and expansion of an effective response to drugs and HIV/AIDS in Malaysia.

In this context, the one element that exemplifies the emerging paradigm shift from compulsory abstinence to voluntary treatment options is the full acceptance of MMT as a legitimate medical treatment for substance dependence. The paradigm shift is also demonstrated by the multiplication of service outlets through which PWUD can access necessary health-care services based on their needs.

In the end, the quality and quantity of MMT services in Malaysia must increase across the board. In particular, more efforts need to be invested in training, registering, accrediting, monitoring and evaluating the next generation of addiction scientists and service providers. The national guidelines, especially as they pertain to MMT dosing, should also be reviewed on a regular basis to accommodate changes in the system and integrate recent developments.

Needle and syringe programmes (NSP)

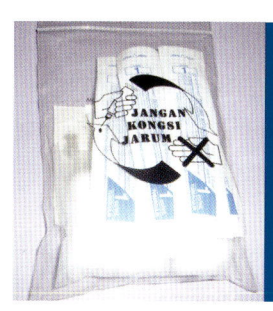

At the beginning of 2010, Malaysia had 240 sites where PWID could access free sterile injecting equipment. The Malaysian NSP services reached 24 999 PWID in 2010, surpassing a target of 15 000 PWID. A total of 2.5 million needles and syringes were distributed in 2009, with a national rate of return of used injecting equipment recorded at 65% (1.6 million needles and syringes). Table 3 provides an overview of the reach of the NSP programme since its inception in 2006.

Table 3: Number of registered NSP clients compared with national targets, 2006–2010 (June)

Year	2006	2007	2008	2009	2010
Target (cumulative)	1 200	7 200	10 800	13 000	15 000
Registered clients (annual)	4 357	2 301	5 572	6 147	6 216
Total clients (cumulative)	4 357	6 658	12 230	18 377	24 999

As in the case of MMT, scale-up of NSPs proceeded rapidly and, in this case, reached the targets set for 2009. Though coverage remains below the ultimate target of reaching 60% of PWID in Malaysia, current targets are being met and expansion of NSP services is proceeding. At inception, only NGOs were delivering NSPs through outreach and DIC-based services. Figure 3 highlights the current active NSP sites operated by NGOs across Malaysia. In 2008, the Government of Malaysia decided to deliver NSP services through local health centres and initiated such services in six centres. At the beginning of 2010, 22 such health centres were implementing NSPs and it is planned to have at least 73 NSPs in government-operated health centres by June 2010. It should also be noted that clinic-based NSP services are offered in parallel with MMT services.

In compliance with the *Needle and syringe exchange programme standard operating policy and guideline*, where NSPs are operating, PWID have access to primary health-care services, referral services for MMT and ART, as well as information and education about HIV prevention and treatment conveying harm reduction and health protection messages, and promoting voluntary counselling and testing and condom use.[17,23] (Condom promotion and use are detailed in a later section, *Sexual transmission among PWUD*.) Through direct observation and analysis of reported data, NSP service providers have indicated that needle-sharing, the driver of HIV

---

23 Power R. *Malaysian needle syringe exchange programme monitoring*. Kuala Lumpur, WHO, 2009.

Figure 3: NGO-operated NSP sites in Malaysia (Malaysian AIDS Council [MAC], 2010)

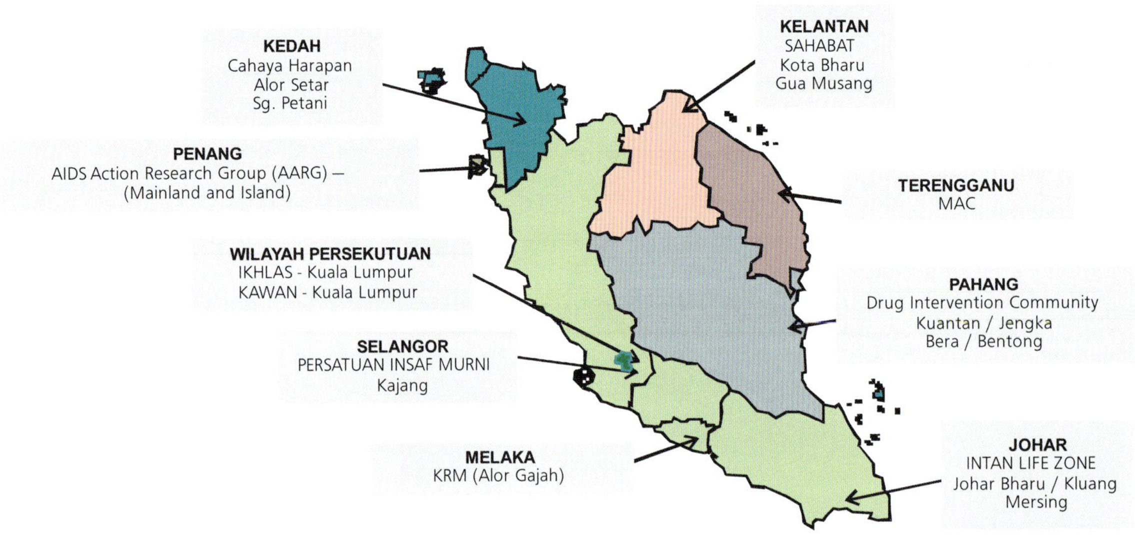

KEDAH
Cahaya Harapan
Alor Setar
Sg. Petani

KELANTAN
SAHABAT
Kota Bharu
Gua Musang

PENANG
AIDS Action Research Group (AARG) —
(Mainland and Island)

TERENGGANU
MAC

WILAYAH PERSEKUTUAN
IKHLAS - Kuala Lumpur
KAWAN - Kuala Lumpur

PAHANG
Drug Intervention Community
Kuantan / Jengka
Bera / Bentong

SELANGOR
PERSATUAN INSAF MURNI
Kajang

MELAKA
KRM (Alor Gajah)

JOHAR
INTAN LIFE ZONE
Johar Bharu / Kluang
Mersing

transmission among PWID, had been reduced.[7] However, despite the possibility of accessing counselling and education services, several stakeholders have pointed out important quality issues, similar to those underlined in the context of the MMT services, whereby existing staff face considerable challenges while trying to meet the demand for services, and are ill-prepared and undertrained to deliver such services.

Sterile injecting equipment is readily available and free of charge at NSP sites. NSP clients are currently being provided with a kit containing four needles, four syringes, 16 cotton balls and 16 alcohol swabs. Although the *Needle syringe exchange programme standard operating policy and guideline* still promotes an exchange of sterile versus used injecting equipment on a one-to-one basis,[24] in practice, PWID are provided with one kit per person per visit.

Based on the results and conclusions of the *Review and evaluation on harm reduction programme in Malaysia* commissioned by WHO,[19] and a workshop report on *Expansion of the harm reduction programme*,[17] several elements of good practice can be highlighted beyond the rapid scale-up of services and diversification of NSP access points.

Recent reports indicate that NSP services are sensitive to clients' needs and deployed over an effective network of organizations and partners, which supports mutual learning and sharing of experiences. This level of cooperation and collaboration

---

24 National Task Force on Harm Reduction. *Needle syringe exchange programme standard operating policy and guidelines*. Kuala Lumpur, Ministry of Health, 2006. Available at: http://www.mac.org.my/v2/wp-content/uploads/attachment/NSEPStdSOP(R).pdf (accessed on 02 March 2011).

is also reflected in programme management efforts, which are integrated with and guided by on-the-ground efforts. Collaboration between government agencies and civil society groups, particularly with NGOs coordinated through MAC, has been stable and productive; support to NGOs has been consistent and existing levels of transparency have facilitated oversight by government agencies.

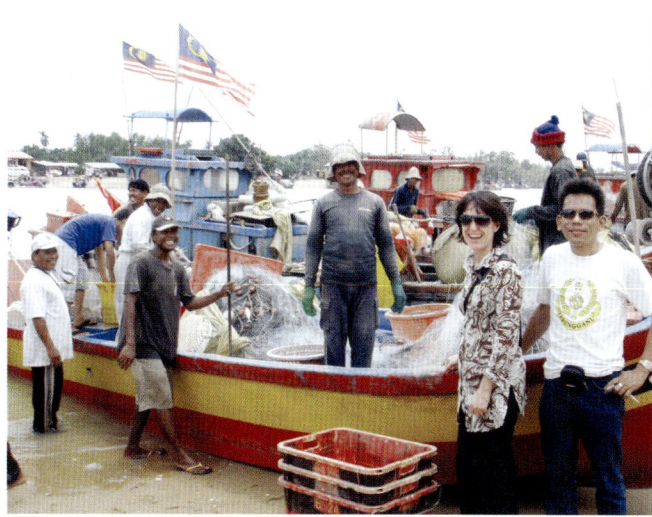

Stakeholders generally agreed that the resources needed for effective programme roll-out were available and adequate.[19] Out of the RM 21 million earmarked for the national harm reduction programme in 2009, RM six million was invested in NSPs. However, stakeholders have repeatedly pointed out that the current system, though financially healthy, requires more effective human resources to meet the demand for services.

To offset the need for trained staff, NGOs have generally invested in empowering PWID from among their clients to undertake the roles of outreach workers and peer educators. Each outreach worker is given an identity card for the purpose of delivering services. The promotion of PWID in strategic implementation roles has greatly contributed to the success of NSPs in Malaysia. A mentoring system along with criteria for employment was put in place to provide support and encourage the development of capacity of PWID. Indeed, there is a general consensus in Malaysia that working with PWID facilitates access to hard-to-reach and hidden vulnerable populations.

In terms of M&E, NSPs operating in Malaysia are coordinated through MAC, which has the ultimate responsibility of reporting back to the MOH. The system in place is effective according to the majority of stakeholders and the *Needle and syringe exchange programme pilot project monitoring and evaluation manual* is a useful tool produced by the NTFHR in 2006, which provides a practical framework to guide further expansion and reporting of NSP activities.[25] In addition, compliance with the *Needle syringe exchange programme standard operating policy and guidelines* is being tracked in existing M&E frameworks with high levels of satisfaction among the majority of stakeholders.

---

25 National Task Force on Harm Reduction. *Needle and syringe exchange programme pilot project monitoring and evaluation manual.* Kuala Lumpur, MOH, 2006.

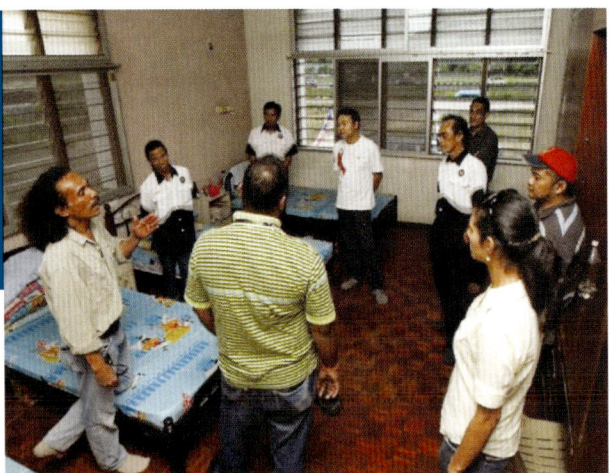

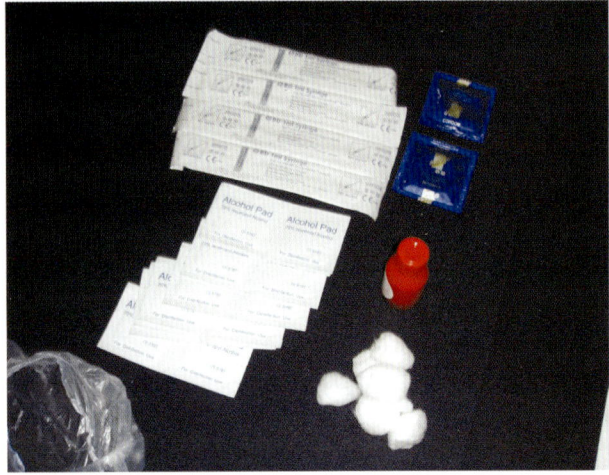

It is easy to conclude that Malaysia's NSPs have incorporated several elements of good practice. In particular, the rapid scale-up of services and expansion of coverage to meet national targets, along with significant financial investments by the government in the national programme, testifies to the existence of high-level commitment and dedicated staff on the frontlines. In addition, the diversity of NSP access points as well as their growing integration with other health and social care services demonstrates that a sophisticated health systems approach was put in place to scale up NSPs, in parallel with MMT services, primary health care, health education and referral networks. PWUD have been empowered to take an active role in the delivery of essential and much-needed services, and have been provided official licence by the authorities to contribute to the success of the response. This represents just one of the examples of effective partnerships that sustain the response in Malaysia – between government agencies undertaking health and law enforcement activities, between government agencies and civil society groups, and between civil society groups and PWUD and other most-at-risk populations (MARPs).

Despite a long history of resistance to NSP from the Malaysian government, the recent integration of NSP into more mainstream health systems such as the local health clinics now confirms the full acceptance of harm reduction as the paradigm of choice to respond to the HIV epidemic in the country. In the context of promotion of voluntary treatment options over total abstinence, implementation practices in the majority of NGO-operated NSPs indicates that the one-to-one exchange has been relaxed to meet existing needs. As such, it is generally recognized that the immediate objectives must concentrate on meeting client needs in terms of health promotion over the ultimate objective of total abstinence.

Antiretroviral treatment (ART) for people who use drugs (PWUD)

At the end of 2009, approximately 35% of PLHIV who needed ART were accessing it, representing 9962 PLHIVs of an estimated 26 722 in need of treatment.[8,16,26] At the end of 2007, a total of about 13 080 PLHIV required ART. However, at the end of 2008, PWID represented less than 25% of those accessing ART, despite the fact that over 70% of PLHIV are current or recovering PWUD.[8,27] Table 4 provides an overview of the rapid expansion of ART access since 2003.

Table 4: Number of PLHIV accessing ART, 2003–2009[8,17,]*

Year	2003	2007	2008	2009
Number of PLHIV accessing ART	1710	6203	8200	9962

*2009 data provided by Dr Fazidah, MOH (personal communication with Pascal Tanguay)

The Malaysian government's commitment to the *National strategic plan on HIV/AIDS 2006–2010* included the allocation of RM 500 million (USD 143 million) over the five-year duration of the Plan.[5] This translates to RM 100 million (approximately USD 28 million) per year to fund government and nongovernment HIV prevention, care and support programmes. This financial support envelope provides for the delivery of ART to 10 000 PLHIV[4] and implies that 2010 targets have almost been met, falling short by just 38 individuals.

In addition to practically meeting targets, it should be noted that existing health systems in place across Malaysia – the networks of antenatal care clinics and local health clinics in rural and urban settings, for example – are well developed and well resourced. Their effectiveness in reaching out to the general population across Malaysia is increasing. The further integration of ART delivery in such existing service networks, as well as with MMT service outlets, has also been noted as a success, where MMT services have been reported to increase ART adherence among PWID.[28] Further expansion of

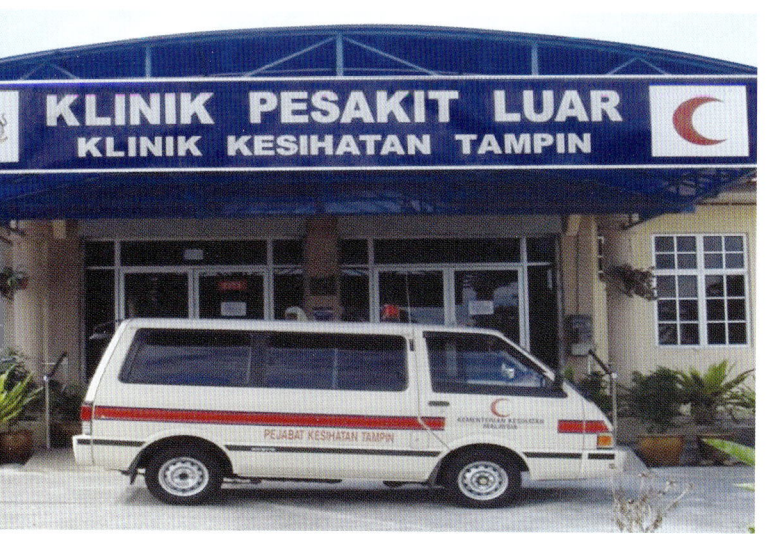

---

26 WHO. *World health statistics 2009*. Geneva, WHO, 2010.
27 Reid G, Kamarulzaman A, Sran SK. Malaysia and harm reduction: the challenges and responses. *International Journal of Drug Policy*, 2006, 18:136–140.
28 Kamarulzaman A. Impact of HIV prevention programs on drug users in Malaysia. *Journal of Acquired Immune Deficiency Syndromes*, 2009, 52:S17–S19.

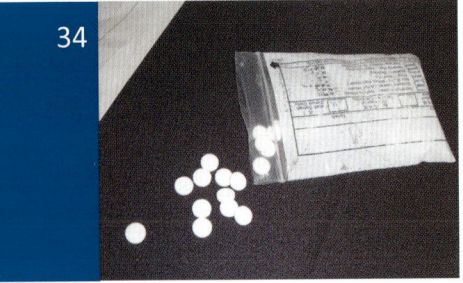

ART delivery in closed settings is proceeding apace as well, with 10 drug treatment centres delivering ART to approximately 110 PLHIV and 15 prisons catering to the needs of incarcerated PLHIV in closed settings.

The mainstay of ART delivery in Malaysia is grounded in provision through family medical specialists. At the end of 2009, there were a total of 170 family medical specialists, of whom 126 had undergone training in HIV treatment.

It is important to recognize the elements of good practice that have become firmly intertwined with the delivery of ART in Malaysia. Where treatment is being delivered, ART has been effective and considered to meet high-quality standards by international experts and local service providers as well as clients. Though the pace of expansion of the ART delivery network has been slower than the expansion of harm reduction services, there has nonetheless been significant expansion in ART provision, even among PWUD.

In that respect, it is critical that further ART delivery capacity be developed at the national level through existing as well as innovative mechanisms if coverage is to increase. In addition, ART initiation criteria should be revised as part of an effort to develop an updated standard operating procedure (SOP) for ART, with a special chapter on ART delivery among PWUD. Just as importantly, further efforts need to be invested in tackling stigma and discrimination, especially among health service providers, in order to facilitate access to essential medicines among MARPs.

Figure 4. Number of PLHIV accessing ART, 2003–2009

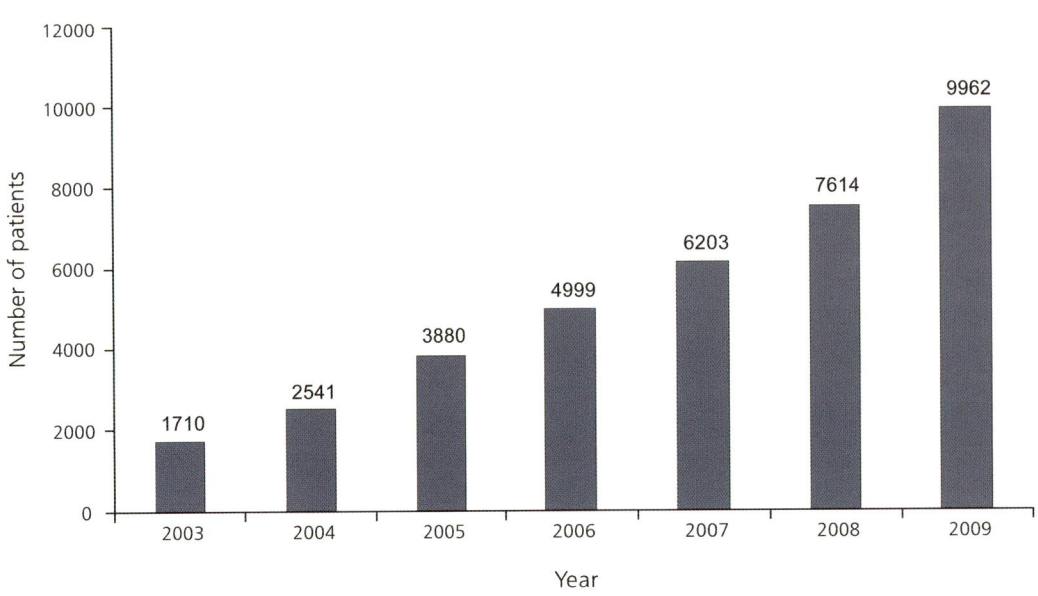

Note: End 2009 – 541 paediatric cases on ART

Sexual transmission among people who use drugs (PWUD)

Although Malaysia's HIV/AIDS epidemic has largely been driven by injecting drug use, recent trends indicate a major increase in transmission through heterosexual sex, which now accounts for approximately 30% of new infections.[29] In an effort to curb sexual transmission among PWID, existing services – MMT, NSPs and to some extent ART provision – have incorporated condom distribution as a complementary service. In 2009, over 93 000 condoms were distributed through MAC (almost twice as many as in 2008), mostly through NSP outreach and DIC-based services.

Although there are very few women and girls who inject drugs (NADA reports that women and girls account for 2.4% of PWUD in Malaysia[30]), MAC has initiated a pilot project targeting their specific needs. The project acknowledges that many women and girls who inject drugs are also involved in sex work. In such a situation where multiple risk factors overlap, the distribution of condoms becomes paramount, along with NSP services. At present, the project delivers health and social care services to approximately 50 female clients, and plans to double the reach. The project operates by hiring female peers to undertake outreach and education activities. In parallel, MOH reports that 284 female clients are registered at MMT service outlets across the country.

Resistance to condom distribution and evidence-based education about sexual and reproductive health for young Malaysians is a clear sign that there are important hurdles that need to be addressed in these areas. In societies heavily influenced by religion, sex is often a taboo, sensitive and contentious subject, because of moral and religious edicts and practices. This situation often reinforces a culture of silence and matters are generally not discussed openly.[30] Some reports indicate that there are strict censorship rules to be observed when discussing condoms or sex in Malaysian media forums as well as in schools.[31]

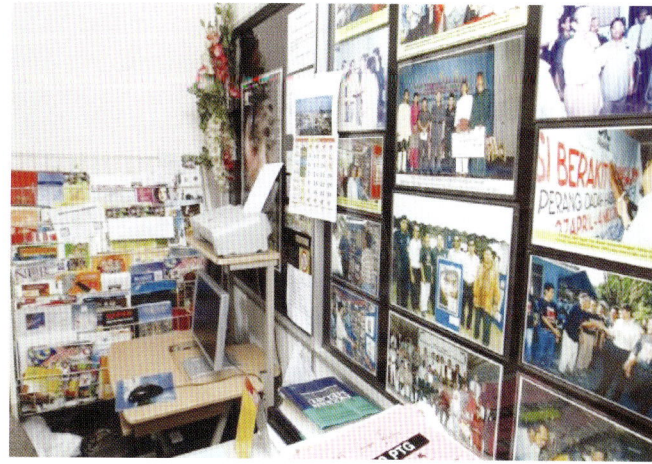

Resistance to effective sex education and promotion of healthy sexual behaviours are based on arguments that discussing a specific behaviour or making commodities available to prevent a consequence of the behaviour may itself lead to increasing the behaviour. This argument has

---

29 "72 percent of AIDS/HIV sufferers in Malaysia are Muslims," says council. *Malay Mail*, 9 June 2010.
30 Bakir Bin HJ Zin A. Assessment of compulsory treatment of people who use drugs in Cambodia, China, Malaysia and Viet Nam: an application of selected human rights principles. Official communication to the Office of the WHO Representative for Brunei Darussalam, Malaysia and Singapore, 9 September 2009.
31 Tai R. *Report on the International Consultation on Risk and responsibilities: male sexual health and HIV in Asia and the Pacific*. 2006. Available at: data.unaids.org/pub/Speech/2006/20060923_sp_pmane_en.pdf (accessed on 02 March 2011).

been a major source of entrenchment around the distribution of needles and syringes across Asia when NSPs were introduced about a decade ago. However, key stakeholders in Malaysia have rapidly agreed that the distribution of needles and syringes does not lead to increased drug use or injecting, and that such a service is necessary to address more pressing objectives.

In the case of sexual transmission, however, the argument that sex education and the distribution of condoms will increase sexual behaviour remains all too common in Malaysia. While key stakeholders have been able to overcome this simple argument with regard to injecting drug use, the belief is entrenched much more deeply with regard to sexual behaviour.

Despite some limitations, the response to sexual transmission of HIV and other blood borne viruses (BBVs) and STIs, especially among PWID, has evolved and continues to build on important successes. For one, the integration of a gendered approach to addressing the needs of PWID is an important step forward and deserves to be sustained and documented further. In addition, the reach of current condom programmes and adaptability of the projects when faced with delivery challenges must be acknowledged as elements of good practice, given the cultural and moral obstacles in the country.

The elements of good practice in the area of NSPs can further enhance condom distribution programmes in Malaysia by addressing popular resistance and opposing arguments. The experience and data generated by NSPs indicate that there are no negative consequences in terms of an increase in drug use and criminal behaviour, and poor health. Further advocacy based on strategies to introduce and scale-up NSPs is urgently needed to tackle resistance to evidence-based sex education and condom distribution.

Such arguments should also be enshrined in an official document to guide and increase the M&E of sex education and condom distribution programmes. Most of the components of the harm reduction programme in Malaysia are guided by SOPs and/or policies. However, in the case of condom distribution and sex education, no such guidelines exist to support implementation. Such a document should also include a specific section on PWUD and other MARPs.

As has been demonstrated for MMT, NSP and ART delivery, the infrastructure of the health-care networks and systems in place across Malaysia is sufficient to rapidly expand condom distribution. Further integration of condom promotion and distribution alongside other health and social care services could significantly strengthen existing mechanisms and expand coverage.

Interventions in closed settings

There are currently 31 prisons in Malaysia as well as at least 16 other detention centres.[13] With approximately 45% of the prison population incarcerated for drug-related crimes,[32] the Malaysian government, particularly under the leadership of MOHA and MOH, decided to implement harm reduction services in closed settings. Since the inception of a pilot MMT project in Pengkalan Chepa prison in April 2008, the MMT programme has expanded and such services were available in 12 prisons at the beginning of 2010.

The MMT programme in Malaysian prisons can significantly reduce the risk of death due to overdose among released PWUD, acknowledging that many continue to use drugs while incarcerated, while those that do not may relapse upon release. The rationale behind the expansion of the prison MMT project is grounded on the objectives of reducing crime and recidivism, and the spread of infectious diseases. There are also indications that MMT in prison settings increases adherence to ART regimens among incarcerated PLHIV.

Though the number of prisons delivering MMT is increasing, the number of clients accessing MMT remains very small.[32] In July 2008, the Pengkalan Chepa prison project had provided MMT to 17 clients since its inception in April 2008; a total of 42 prisoners were enrolled in the prison MMT programme across the pilot project scheme implemented in three institutions in 2008. In January 2009, the project had expanded to cover five prisons.[28]

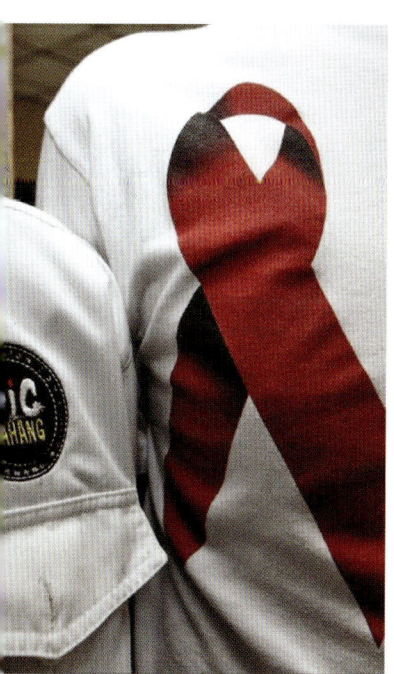

The implementation and scale-up of MMT in prison settings is largely due to effective partnerships and collaboration between the MOH, MOHA and the Prison Department. Staff across participating prisons have become increasingly sensitized to the needs of PWUD and understand that MMT is a medical treatment that can significantly facilitate prison management and operations. Prison guards and authorities have also accepted the assistance of NGOs for various aspects of the MMT programme in prisons. It is also clear that health systems' integration has significantly contributed to the effectiveness and success of this project, as evidenced by the multisectoral nature of the response in prisons.

Harm reduction programmes have recently been initiated in drug rehabilitation centres, particularly MMT and ART for PWUD. As noted earlier, 10 such centres are providing ART to 110 clients. In contrast, MMT was initiated in July 2008 in six centres, covering the needs of 251 clients. The introduction of such health-care

---

32 MOHA. *Drug information 2009*. Kuala Lumpur, Ministry of Home Affairs, 2009.

services for PWUD is part of a strategy to convert drug rehabilitation centres into "cure and care" centres. The new approach, developed under the leadership of NADA, is predicated on the imperative of addressing the needs of PWUD instead of forcing uniform treatment programmes upon them. Between July and December 2010, NADA was operating six such centres in primary hotspots with plans to expand coverage to ten centres in 2011.

The cure and care approach is an important landmark in Malaysia's response to drug use and HIV/AIDS. The objectives and activities of the operational model in drug rehabilitation centres confirm the shift from punitive approaches to harm reduction models. The recent changes also confirm that a new paradigm is emerging, where a variety of treatment options that best meet clients' needs are available for them to choose from within these government-operated institutions. However, despite the introduction of harm reduction services in cure and care centres as well as in drug rehabilitation centres, many stakeholders have highlighted that access to condoms and quality counselling requires urgent attention.

Again, the integration of new models and practices in the existing health-care systems in Malaysia is testimony to high-level leadership, sensible and evidence-based decision-making, strong and effective partnerships, and a commitment to invest necessary resources. Yet, limitations in terms of human resources have been voiced: more staff and capacity are urgently needed to further scale-up and strengthen the cure and care centres. Despite the human resource challenges, existing staff are increasingly professional in terms of documentation and reporting against M&E frameworks, and also more sensitized to the needs of PWUD and the precepts of the addiction sciences.

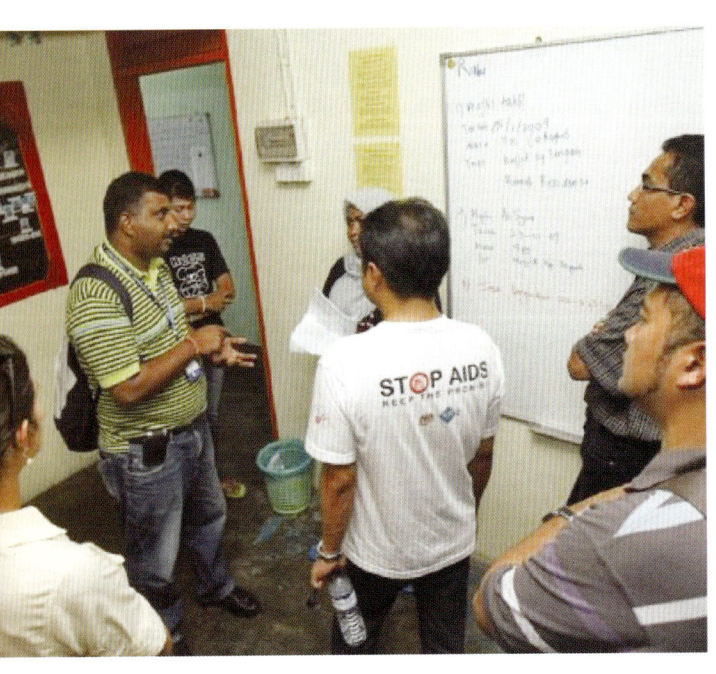

In 2007, MMT was initiated in three NADA-operated aftercare centres. By the end of 2009, all 24 aftercare centres under NADA supervision were delivering MMT along with basic HIV education. The impressive speed with which MMT has been scaled up in such institutions is worth highlighting. However, issues related to the quality of counselling have been repeatedly stressed in the context of aftercare centres.

Effective partnerships between NADA, MOH and University Malaya Medical Centre (UMMC) have been critical in setting up MMT delivery in aftercare centres in Malaysia. More recently, NGOs have also been invited to work alongside government agencies to provide support in such centres. In effect, the harmonization of care with services available in community settings as well as in prison and drug treatment centres also indicates that delivery of health services across closed settings is part of a broader strategy to integrate health systems.

The presence of aftercare centres undoubtedly facilitates the reintegration of those discharged from closed institutions and also simultaneously increases the possibility of continuity of treatment and sustainability of health-care interventions. The change in attitudes of staff working in such centres is also an important factor in stimulating motivation among clients. With the leadership of NADA promoting an alternative approach focused on providing access to a range of voluntary treatment options, staff in such institutions are likely to adjust their attitudes, as has happened in prison settings.

In conclusion, the elements of good practice in Malaysia's national response to drugs and HIV in closed settings are numerous and important. The rapid scale-up of MMT and ART in prisons, rehabilitation, cure and care centres, and aftercare institutions also demonstrates that the commitment to harm reduction in the country is supported by effective action. In parallel, it is clear that the introduction MMT and ART services has been aligned with existing health systems and integrated to facilitate expansion and minimize costs. The professionalization of staff working in closed settings is also noticeable, where attitudes towards PWUD are changing based on evidence and new strategic directions.

Perhaps one of the most novel and exciting elements of good practice in responding to the needs of PWUD in Malaysia is occurring at the periphery of the national harm reduction programme. At a time when international stakeholders are reviewing the necessity for and effectiveness of drug treatment centres, Malaysia has already reduced its reliance on such systems in favour of community-based approaches. More importantly, the operational model underpinning the operations of drug rehabilitation centres is being transformed, from a compulsory treatment approach to the provision of a range of treatment alternatives to best meet the immediate needs of PWUD.

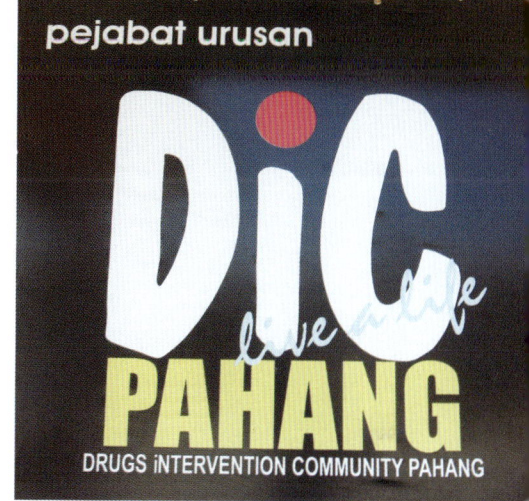

It is here that we can see evidence of a new paradigm shift occurring in Malaysia. Though an important paradigm shift from punitive to harm reduction approaches has already taken place and has been confirmed here and elsewhere, the current transformation of the response to drugs and HIV/AIDS in Malaysia indicates that a new model is emerging. The integration of drug dependence treatment and harm reduction services with HIV prevention, treatment, care and support services places Malaysia in a leadership position compared with neighbouring countries in the Region.

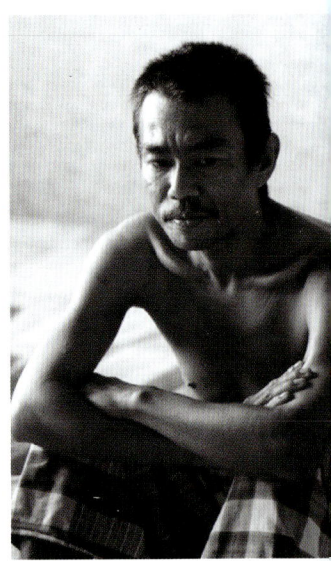

Despite such a leadership position, much remains to be done to effectively prevent the transmission of HIV and other BBVs and STIs in closed settings. Though MMT and ART services are key elements in the WHO comprehensive package of effective interventions for PWID, other services need to be integrated across custodial settings. For example, the introduction of NSPs in closed settings could significantly contribute to a decrease in HIV transmission among PWID. It is also critical that condoms be made available to individuals residing in closed settings in order to prevent sexual transmission of BBVs and STIs.

3 Analysis of cross-cutting themes

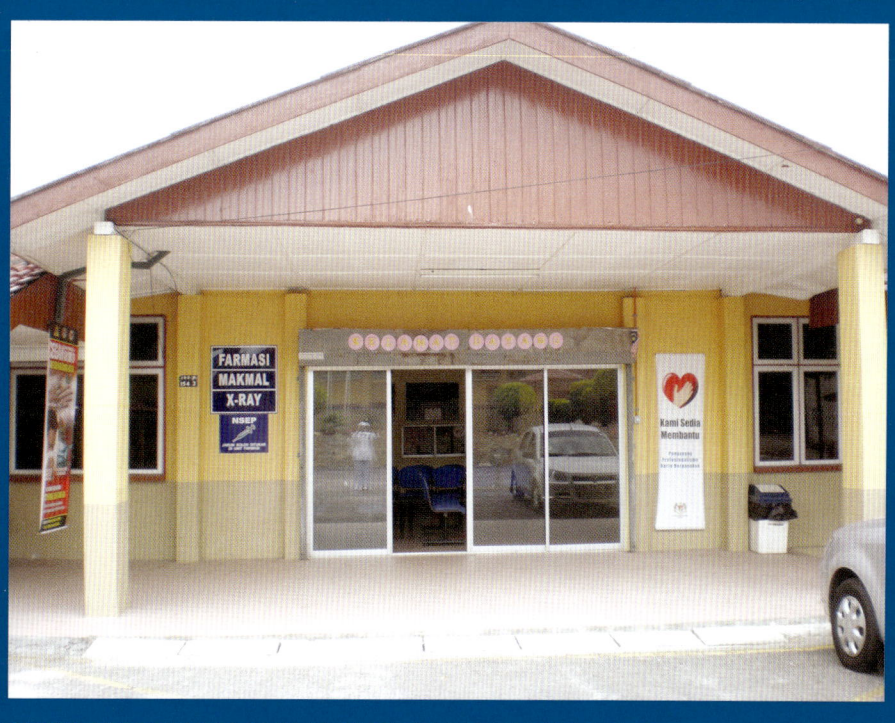

Analysis of cross-cutting themes

As noted above, Malaysia's response to drugs and HIV/AIDS includes many of the core elements of the comprehensive package of effective interventions recommended by WHO to prevent HIV transmission among PWID. It is important to highlight the common elements of good practice across these interventions, as well as the cross-cutting challenges. Some key issues have been underlined under each intervention and this section seeks to analyse those key themes before presenting a concluding overview of good practice elements and recommendations to improve the national response.

The key themes analysed in this section include: communication and advocacy, health systems and human resources, and partnerships and the involvement of civil society and law enforcement. The exploration of these topics based on each intervention in the previous section can now provide insight into existing strengths and challenges.

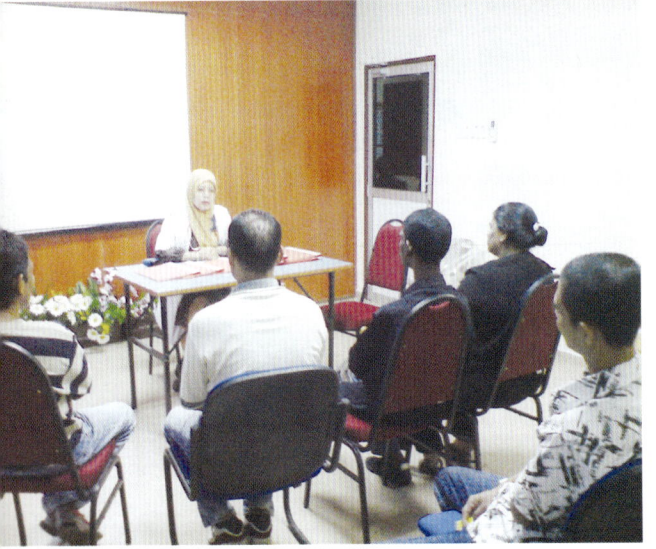

Communication and advocacy

Communication between and among key stakeholders involved in the design, implementation and M&E of the national response to drugs and HIV/AIDS is generally smooth and effective, according to the majority of key stakeholders. This is paralleled by effective advocacy among the same groups. There are reports that the advocacy efforts of medical officers have been critical in scaling up MMT across the country.[27] The heads of key civil society and government agencies have in effect become the leaders of the harm reduction movement, champions internal to the national response. Current leadership in MOH, MOHA and MAC indicate that there is growing alignment of objectives through effective and regular communication in Malaysia.

However, communication and advocacy targeting stakeholders outside the scope of the response have been characterized as weak by many.[17] Recommendations have previously been formulated to address public perception of PWUD in Malaysia. Though increasing numbers of media articles are being published on the achievements of the national harm reduction programme, the vast majority of media reports have reinforced stigma and discrimination against PWUD. Current levels of stigma and discrimination remain high and often pose significant barriers to implementation and service delivery, particularly in the case of NSPs.[17,23,28] It is becoming increasingly important that public perceptions and related stigmatization and discrimination of PWUD be addressed to ensure the success of Malaysia's response to drugs and HIV/AIDS.

This report is intended both for national and Regional audiences, and WHO commits to facilitating the use of this report at both the national and Regional levels. WHO considers this report as an advocacy tool to guide further expansion of the national response to drugs and HIV/AIDS in Malaysia as well as to encourage other governments in Asia to develop and incorporate elements of good practice in their national responses.

To further build on the national and regional strategic communication objectives of this report, WHO encourages Malaysian government agencies, in partnership with civil society representatives, to develop and implement a national communication strategy. The development of such a strategy would be well timed, as key stakeholders are currently discussing the development of the *National strategic plan on HIV/AIDS 2011–2015*. The parallel development of a communication strategy could significantly add value to the national strategic plan on HIV/AIDS while addressing national issues around stigma and discrimination, and increase the Regional visibility of Malaysia's national response to drugs and HIV/AIDS.

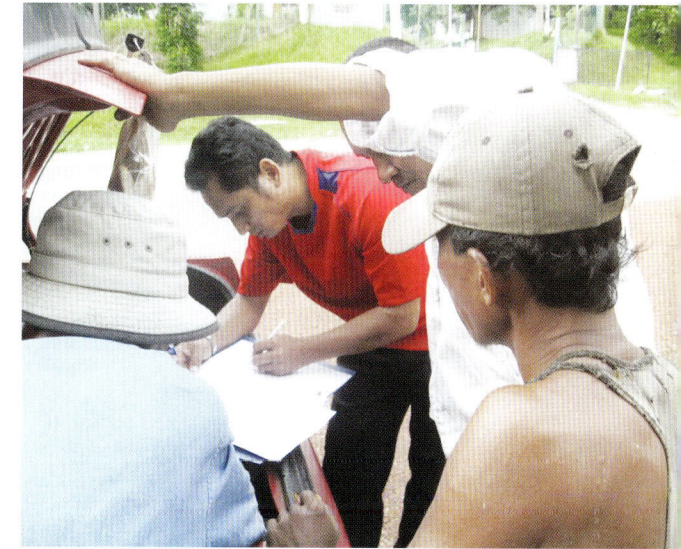

Health systems and human resources

Across the majority of interventions for drugs and HIV in place in Malaysia, those with health service components have been integrated into existing national health systems. At the same time, the integration of harm reduction services has reinforced and strengthened existing service delivery systems. Programmes such as MMT and ART have been facilitated by a strong commitment from the medical community, both in terms of advocacy as well as implementation.

The case of integration of condoms and sex education is particularly challenging in a country where people, especially decision-makers, are heavily influenced by religion. This issue has been highlighted in other countries where the majority of the population is Muslim, where religious attitudes lend a moral value to behaviours, commodities and even words. Though the resistance to harm reduction programmes among religious leaders has been effectively addressed, the resistance to sexual and reproductive health education and services remains strong.

The expansion and integration of harm reduction programmes in mosques is particularly important. Not only does this programme further integrate harm reduction in broader health and social care systems, it also addresses an important caveat of shortage of human resources.

The case of providing counselling services in parallel with other harm reduction services has been highlighted several times but is by no means an exception. The same case has been made for increased human resources and capacity for MMT, ART, NSP and in closed settings, both in government and civil society agencies and organizations.

Partnerships

The number and quality of partnerships forged to support the design, implementation and M&E of the national response to drugs and HIV/AIDS in Malaysia have been to some extent reflected in the analysis of communication strategies and health systems' integration processes. However, it is worth noting here that partnerships between government agencies working on health and drug control, and civil society groups, academia, religious leaders and key leaders have played a critical role in the expansion of harm reduction services. Multisectoral involvement in the response has been characterized by strong buy-in and ownership among virtually all agencies and stakeholders. This has enormously facilitated collaboration as well as built transparent and accountable relationships between all stakeholders across the national response.

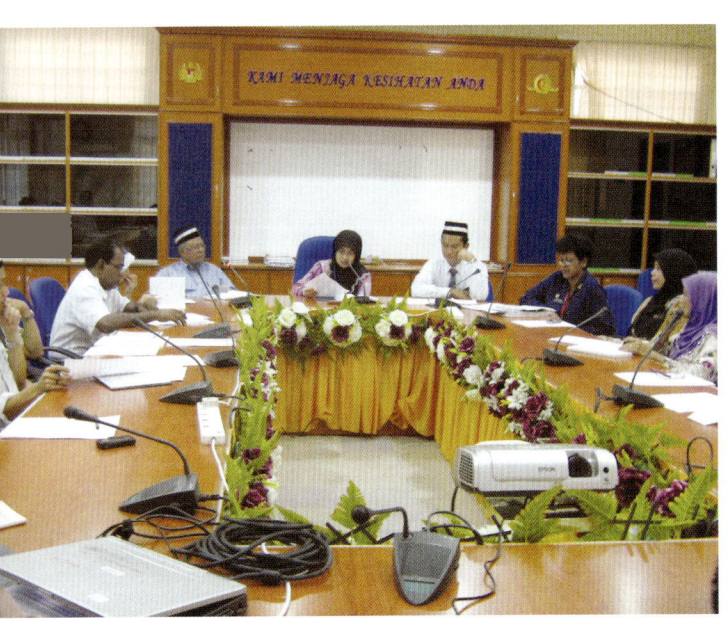

It is worth repeating that in the context of civil society partnerships, MAC plays an important role. MAC's role focuses around the same responsibilities delegated to national AIDS committees in other countries, usually operating under the MOH. MAC therefore enjoys an important role in coordinating the national response and has invested significant resources and energy in the national harm reduction programme. However, despite this role, MAC is not a government agency and therefore often lacks the binding power to stimulate action. Despite these limitations, MAC has learned to operate in ways that stimulate consensus and has developed close working relationships with strategic leaders and decision-makers, an approach well suited to the Malaysian context.

Other civil society agencies such as the Pink Triangle (PT) Foundation also enjoy a high status through the long-standing reputation of delivering quality outputs that are aligned with national objectives. However, compared with other Asian countries, there are very few civil society groups involved in the national response to drugs and HIV/AIDS. This may be due to the perception that existing agencies have filled the harm reduction market niche and that such work attracts similar stigma as that against PWUD in Malaysia.

In addition, though clients are often asked to report on their appreciation of the services they access, their involvement in the design, implementation and M&E of interventions that target them is generally very limited. Services such as MMT and ART are highly medicalized, leaving the involvement of PWUD almost confined to implementation of NSPs. Despite this situation, civil society representatives are currently working on setting up the Malaysian Network of People who Use Drugs, an organization operated by PWUD to increase the meaningful involvement of Malaysian PWUD in the national response.

In addition to the involvement of civil society, it is critical to reflect on the meaningful role of law enforcement in the national response. In recognition of the critical role of law enforcement in the response to drugs and HIV/AIDS in Malaysia, the composition of the NHRTF includes seats for representatives from both NADA and the Royal Malaysian Police Force.[28] This high-level coordination is critical for the alignment of objectives, and delivery of and effective access to health services among PWUD.

Strengthening the capacity of local law enforcement officers as well as prison staff has been addressed through several workshops convened by Malaysian authorities,[28] while a harm reduction module has been integrated in the Royal Malaysian Police Force Training Academy. One such national workshop was delivered by the International Drug Policy Consortium in December 2009, which provided senior members of three law enforcement agencies with information and skills to use strategies that avoid breaches in human rights standards or involve widespread or discriminatory arrests of PWUD. The workshop also provided concrete opportunities for meaningful involvement of law enforcement in partnerships to support harm reduction and simultaneously achieve drug control objectives. One critical topic addressed in the workshop was the need to ensure harmonization between "management cops" and "street cops".

However, additional training for law enforcement and prison staff is required, and has been systematically recommended by various stakeholders.[17,23,28] Run-ins, mishaps and raids compromising health service delivery, especially at NGO-operated facilities, continue to be reported by PWUD and those who facilitate service access, despite ongoing trainings. Additional training and sensitization are urgently needed to align high-level decisions with practice on the frontlines.

Overall, the response to drugs and HIV/AIDS in Malaysia is part of a joint effort involving committed and diverse stakeholders, all of whom share roles and responsibilities. The involvement of law enforcement and civil society groups also demonstrates that the national response has rapidly matured and operates through the willing participation of all relevant stakeholders.

Tampin District Health Services

WHO's *Country Cooperation Strategy 2009–2013* for Malaysia presents the Tampin District Health Centre as a model of good practice in harm reduction service delivery.[33] The Tampin District Health Centre is one of many such centres that operate across Malaysia, mostly in rural areas. District health centres often represent the first point of access to health services for the population.

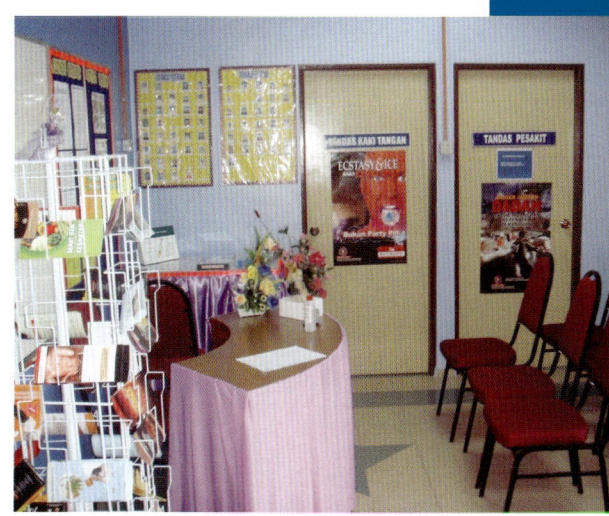

In July 2005, the Tampin District Health Centre initiated ART services to meet the needs of a growing number of PLHIV in the community. As the health centre became increasingly aware that most PLHIV in the area in and around Tampin District were contracting HIV through injecting drug use, the health centre authorities in partnership with several community and government stakeholders agreed to initiate MMT delivery as well. The MMT programme was thus started in 2006. Beyond the important services provided to PWUD in Tampin District, clients of the MMT programme soon informed the authorities that more needed to be done to meet their needs. Acknowledging this, in July 2008, NSPs were set up in five health centres, operating in parallel with ART and MMT programmes. Today, all health clinics across Tampin District provide MMT and NSP services, as well as outreach.

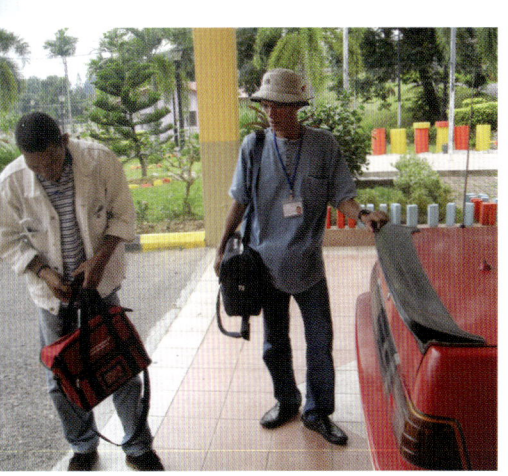

In its MMT programme and in line with the national guidelines, the Tampin District Health Centre has initiated a system to provide clients with a limited and closely monitored number of take-away doses. However, the system of take-away doses implemented in the clinic is based on creating incentives among PWUD, rather than delivering sanctions and punishment. Clients are rewarded with a number of points for participating in clinic activities and they can "buy" take-away doses from the service providers.

Both the delivery of MMT and the NSP in Tampin District could not have happened without the dedicated leadership of key individuals. In addition,

....

33   WHO. *Malaysia Country Cooperation Strategy 2009–2013*. Manila, WHO WPRO/Ministry of Health Malaysia, 2010.

the sustainability of the project is guaranteed by the meaningful involvement of health professionals, local government authorities, religious leaders, local law enforcement officials as well as the clients themselves. All these groups are represented in a District Harm Reduction Committee that oversees and monitors the performance of the projects. WHO reports that improvements in the quality of life, high retention rates, and prevention of HIV, other BBVs and STI have been measured since the implementation of the harm reduction services.[33]

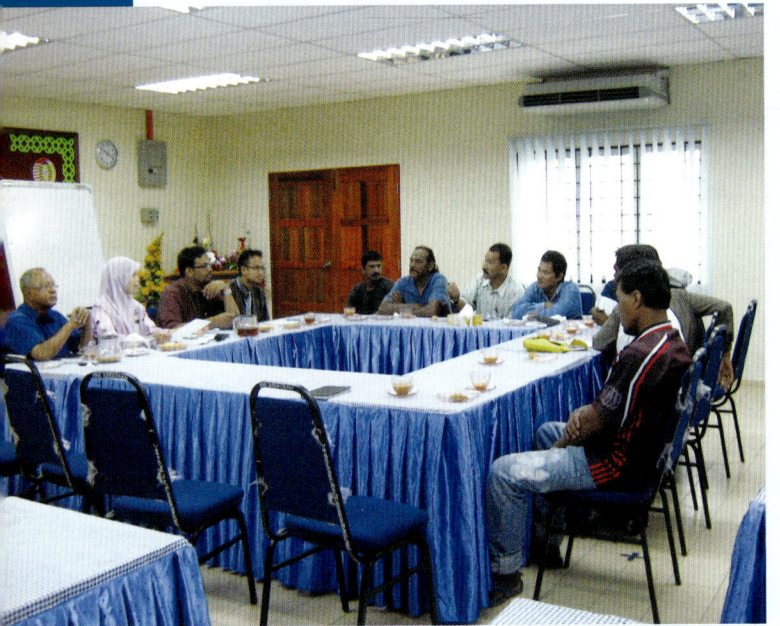

Another key to the success achieved in Tampin District has been the integration of harm reduction services with the existing health systems in place. The network of district health centres across Malaysia is a common model in Asia whereby low-threshold health services can be accessed easily and within a reasonable travel distance. The authorities in Tampin District quickly recognized that such integration would facilitate service delivery and, with support from MOH and NADA, responded to a wide range of needs among PWUD in the area.

4 Conclusions and Recommendations

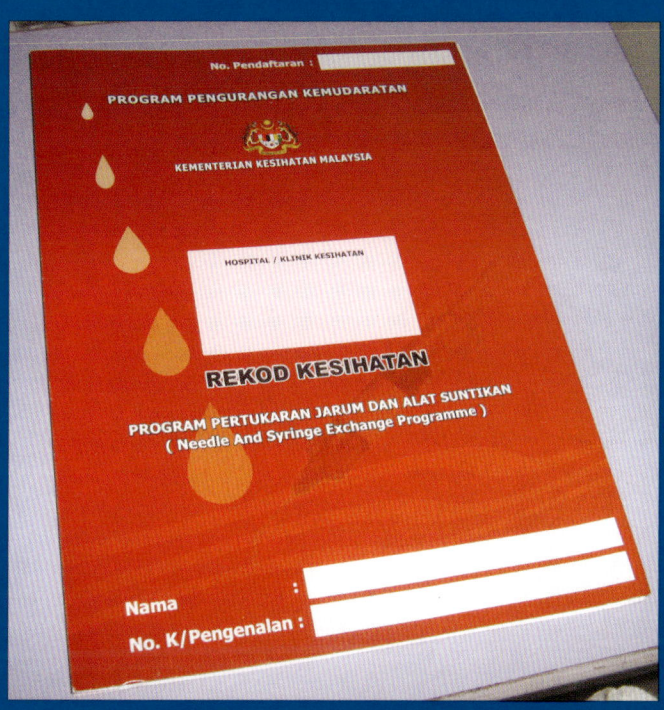

Conclusions and Recommendations

This report has sought to highlight elements of good practice in Malaysia's national response to drugs and HIV/AIDS as well as identify gaps to further improve the response. This has been done by providing an overview of the scale-up process, modalities, partnerships, capacity, resources and M&E structures for a range of interventions to prevent HIV transmission among PWUD. An analysis of cross-cutting issues has further highlighted some important elements of success as well as gaps in the response. A summary of these elements is provided below, organized by individual interventions as well as across cross-cutting themes.

Conclusions: elements of good practice

Methadone maintenance therapy (MMT)

- Rapid scale-up of free MMT services over the past five years across the country;

- Detectable impact on PWUD's lifestyles; higher employment rates among clients and increased adherence to ART;

- Multiplication of a variety of service access points, including across closed settings, mosques, government hospitals and district health clinics;

- Documentation of client satisfaction at service access points;

- Deployment of a national policy and SOP to guide implementation, reporting and evaluation of projects;

- Development and implementation of a national MMT provider registration and accreditation system along with capacity-building modules to scale-up human resource capacity;

- Allocation of significant resources from national budgets;

- Integration of MMT in existing health systems as well as in a comprehensive package of interventions to prevent HIV, BBV and STI transmission;

- Collaboration through genuine and honest partnerships among government agencies leading public health and drug control activities, and civil society, religious leaders and medical professionals;

- High-level commitment and leadership from key agencies and individuals; and

- Deployment of a national M&E framework to track progress, success and challenges.

Needle and syringe programmes (NSPs)

- Rapid scale-up of free NSP services over the past five years across the country, mostly through civil society efforts;

- Recent involvement of government agencies, through district health clinics among others, in NSP delivery;

- Detectable impact on reducing needle and syringe sharing among PWUD;

- Meeting national targets set through the National strategic plan on HIV/AIDS 2006–2010;

- Hiring of PWUD to work in NSP projects as peer outreach workers and educators;

- Licensed protection of outreach workers and peer educators operating NSPs through the provision of official identification cards;

- Deployment of a national SOP to guide implementation modalities, and reporting and evaluation of projects;

- Integration of NSPs in existing health systems as well as in a comprehensive package of interventions to prevent HIV, BBV and STI transmission;

- Recognized to meet client needs at health service access points;

- Collaboration through genuine and honest partnerships among government agencies, particularly in terms of the roles and responsibilities delegated to MAC;

- Allocation of significant resources from national budgets;

- High-level commitment and leadership from key agencies and individuals; and

- Demonstrated will and interest in reinforcing harm reduction approaches while building access to a wide range of health-care services to meet PWUD's needs.

Antiretroviral treatment (ART)

- Considerable scale-up of ART over the past 15 years across the country;

- Meeting national targets set through the National strategic plan on HIV/AIDS 2006–2010;

- Multiplication of a variety of service access points, including across closed settings, as well as government hospitals and district health clinics;

- Allocation of significant resources from national budgets;
- High-level commitment and leadership from key agencies and individuals; and
- Integration of ART in existing health systems as well as in a comprehensive package of interventions to prevent HIV, BBV and STI transmission.

Sexual transmission among PWUD

- Substantial and continued scale-up of condom distribution across the country;
- Demonstrated capacity to adapt programmes to meet client needs; and
- Budding integration of gender issues in the national response to drugs and HIV/AIDS.

Interventions in closed settings

- Rapid scale-up of free MMT and ART in closed settings – including prisons, cure and care centres, as well as aftercare centres;
- Observable impact on reducing the risk of overdose upon release, increasing the possibility of continuity of care among PWUD;
- Collaboration through genuine and honest partnerships among government agencies leading public health and drug control activities, and the prison department, civil society and medical professionals;
- Integration of ART and NSPs in existing health systems in prisons and cure and care centres, as well as in a comprehensive package of interventions to prevent HIV, BBV and STI transmission;
- Visible professionalization of staff and officials working in closed settings;
- Rapid transformation of compulsory drug rehabilitation centres focusing on abstinence into cure and care centres with a wide range of treatment and care options to meet PWUD's needs;
- Significantly reduced reliance on drug rehabilitation centres and compulsory treatment;
- Increased interest in and reliance on community justice mechanisms and diversion from criminal systems to health systems;

- High-level commitment and leadership from key agencies and individuals; and
- Demonstrated will and interest in reinforcing harm reduction approaches while building access to a wide range of health-care services to meet PWUD's needs.

Communication and advocacy

- Excellent internal communication between stakeholders involved in the response to drugs and HIV/AIDS leading to effective advocacy.

Health systems and human resources

- Integration of harm reduction services in a comprehensive package of interventions to prevent and treat HIV/AIDS among PWUD, made available through a variety of service access points and settings;
- Integration of the components of the national harm reduction programme in existing national health systems; and
- Significant achievements in scaling up the national harm reduction programme with current human resources and capacity.

Partnerships

- National harm reduction programme implemented by a wide range of stakeholders from various sectors with strong ownership across the stakeholder spectrum;
- Important and increasing contributions from civil society groups in the national response to drugs and HIV/AIDS;
- Deployment of an SOP to oversee and facilitate law enforcement interventions at service delivery sites; and
- Increasing interest in and motivation for further integration of harm reduction components in the national training for law enforcement officials and officers.

The report also proposes that a second paradigm shift is taking place in Malaysia, moving from a compulsory abstinence model to a model based on voluntary access to a wide range of treatment options. Evidence has been provided here to indicate that such a shift may have been initiated very recently. Of particular importance is the recent directives issued by NADA, essentially converting compulsory drug rehabilitation centres into voluntary cure and care centres that cater to the needs of PWUD through a wide range of effective interventions.

The shift can also be reflected in an increasing range of available health and social care services as well as their integration with other health systems already in place in Malaysia. The provision of MMT and ART in one location, particularly in closed settings, also lends weight to the proposition of an emerging paradigm. With an expanded range of such institutions providing health and social care services for PWUD – whether they be delivered through hospitals, district health clinics, NGO-operated DICs, prisons and other closed institutions, or mosques – access to health service options in Malaysia has been systematically increasing. The range of services offered at each site is also increasing rapidly, from virtually no harm reduction services in 2005 to a full-fledged national programme within five years. This emerging paradigm is an important element of good practice, resulting in a decreased reliance on compulsory treatment centres as well as marking a more sensitized and evidence-based response to the needs of PWUD.

Although this success is important and deserves to be highlighted nationally and regionally, the further development and expansion of the Malaysian response to drugs and HIV/AIDS faces important challenges. Through the analysis in this report, several elements for improvement have been identified. A list of summary recommendations is given below.

Recommendations

Methadone maintenance therapy (MMT)

- Build the capacity of existing service delivery staff and develop incentives to attract additional qualified human resources to expand service delivery.

- In parallel, address the growing demand for MMT services among PWUD and reduce the waiting time for accessing MMT while increasing coverage among PWUD.

- Involve GPs in the delivery of MMT services by addressing issues such as capacity and time management.

- Create additional spaces for the meaningful involvement of civil society groups, particularly PWUD, in the design, delivery and M&E of MMT programmes.

- Increase the quality of counselling through capacity building, exposure and incentives to attract qualified staff.

- Work towards an overall increase in MMT dosages to comply with international guidelines.

- Synchronize and consolidate reporting mechanisms into one official national structure.

- Revise MMT policies and SOPs to adapt to emerging realities and practices.

Needle and syringe programmes (NSPs)

- Build the capacity of existing service delivery staff and develop incentives to attract additional qualified human resources to expand service delivery.

- In parallel, rapidly develop and implement effective support mechanisms for peer outreach workers and educators such as quality counselling, fair market-value salaries and relapse prevention measures.

- Rapidly and officially address the issue of continuing law enforcement raids at service delivery sites, especially where NGO-operated projects are being implemented.

- Revise the SOP for NSP to adapt to emerging realities and practices, especially to address one-to-one exchange of sterile injecting equipment.

- Harmonize laws and policies to avoid criminalization of essential health services.

Antiretroviral treatment (ART)

- Rapidly increase access to ART among PWUD, in particular, by revising induction criteria that discriminate against PWUD.

- Build the capacity of existing service delivery staff and develop incentives to attract additional qualified human resources to expand service delivery.

- Involve GPs in the delivery of ART services by building capacity and providing exposure to other service sites in the Region.

Sexual transmission among PWUD

- Urgently scale-up condom distribution for MARPs, particularly among PWUD in government-operated closed settings.

- Rapidly address the practice of detaining individuals carrying condoms for potential solicitation and generate incentives for more consistent condom use.

- Establish partnerships with media agencies to disseminate non-discriminatory messages about drug dependence and HIV prevention to address stigmatizing public perceptions.

- Ensure that evidence-based sexual and reproductive health information is integrated in the primary and high school curriculum.

- Rapidly form partnerships between harm reduction advocates and sexual and reproductive health advocates to disseminate the strategies used to integrate NSPs in the national harm reduction programme in order to support condom distribution.

- Given that health systems already exist to support effective condom distribution and evidence-based sexual and reproductive health services, ensure that expansion of such programmes are integrated with the existing mechanisms in place.

- Develop and deploy an SOP to guide implementation of a condom distribution programme across the country.

Interventions in closed settings

- Continue to reduce the number of compulsory drug treatment centres and, in parallel, facilitate access to free outpatient evidence-based drug treatment.

- Build the capacity of existing service delivery staff and develop incentives to attract additional qualified human resources to expand service delivery.

- In parallel, rapidly increase the coverage of available harm reduction components, particularly MMT and ART, across prisons, cure and care and aftercare centres.

- Urgently ensure access to condoms, sterile injecting equipment and quality counselling across closed settings.

Communication and advocacy

- Develop strategies and activities to address stigma and discrimination towards PWUD and initiatives for the management of public perception.

CONCLUSIONS AND RECOMMENDATIONS

- Collaborate with media agencies and representatives to disseminate non-discriminatory messages relating to PWUD and HIV prevention.

- Rapidly develop and integrate a national communications strategy in parallel with the emerging national strategic plan.

Health systems and human resources

- Across interventions, urgently work towards and invest in the expansion of significant human resources and workforce development, in particular for counsellors, medical officers and law enforcement officers.

Partnerships

- Create opportunities for the meaningful involvement of PWUD in the design, implementation and M&E of the national harm reduction programme.

- Increase and reinforce capacity-building programmes for law enforcement officers.

- Rapidly and officially address the issue of continuing law enforcement raids at service delivery sites, especially where NGO-operated projects are being implemented.

- Harmonize laws and policies to avoid criminalization of essential health services.